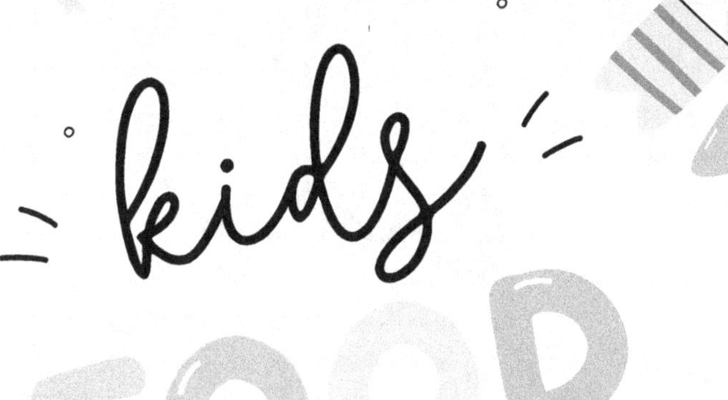

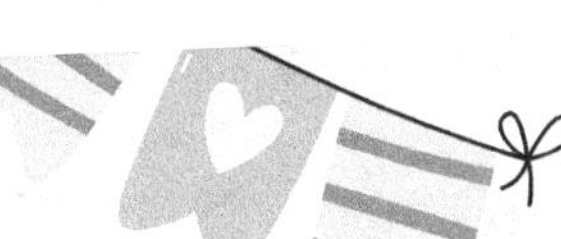

BREAKFAST

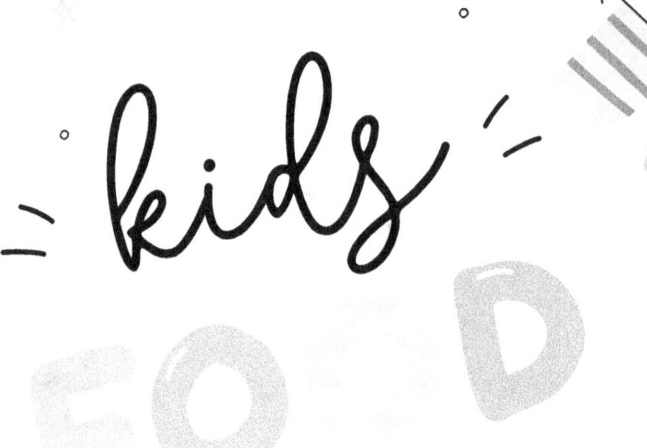

kids FOOD

SNACKS

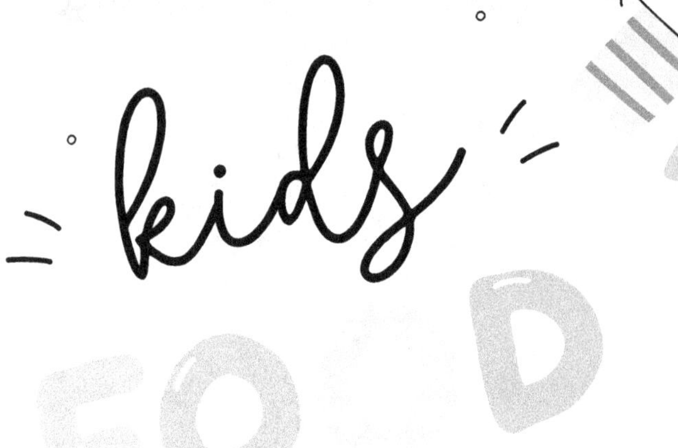

DINNER

70. Spaghetti with Meatballs ... 75
71. Chicken and Broccoli Stir-Fry ... 76
72. Baked Salmon with Green Beans ... 77
73. Veggie Lasagna ... 78
74. Beef Tacos with Avocado ... 79
75. Chicken Alfredo Pasta ... 80
76. Baked Ziti with Ricotta ... 81
77. Grilled Chicken with Quinoa ... 82
78. Shepherd's Pie ... 83
79. Veggie and Cheese Pizza ... 84
80. Shrimp Fried Rice ... 85
81. Stuffed Bell Peppers ... 86
82. BBQ Chicken Drumsticks ... 87
83. Veggie Frittata ... 88
84. Baked Tilapia with Lemon ... 89
85. Chicken and Veggie Skewers ... 90
86. Beef and Bean Chili ... 91
87. Veggie Stir-Fry with Tofu ... 92
88. Grilled Cheese and Tomato Soup ... 93
89. Chicken Pot Pie ... 94
90. Pork Chops with Mashed Potatoes ... 95
91. Veggie Enchiladas ... 96
92. Meatloaf with Mixed Veggies ... 97
93. Teriyaki Chicken with Rice

kids FOOD

BAKING

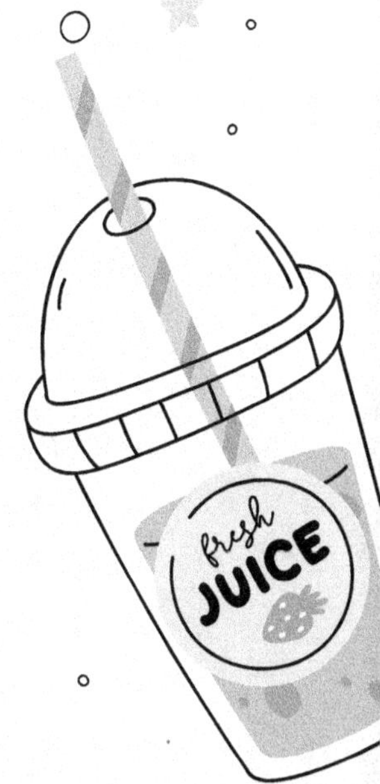

1. Pancakes with Fresh Berries

Ingredients:
- 1 cup all-purpose flour
- 2 tablespoons sugar
- 2 teaspoons baking powder
- 1/2 teaspoon salt
- 1 cup milk
- 2 tablespoons unsalted butter, melted
- 1 egg
- 1 cup fresh berries (such as blueberries, raspberries, or strawberries)

Equipment:
- Mixing bowl
- Whisk
- Griddle or non-stick skillet
- Spatula

Directions:
1. In a mixing bowl, whisk together the flour, sugar, baking powder, and salt.
2. In a separate bowl, whisk together the milk, melted butter, and egg.
3. Pour the wet ingredients into the dry ingredients and stir just until combined (do not overmix).
4. Heat a griddle or non-stick skillet over medium heat. Lightly grease the surface.
5. Scoop about 1/4 cup of batter onto the hot surface and cook for 2-3 minutes, or until bubbles start to form on the surface.
6. Flip the pancake and cook for an additional 1-2 minutes, or until golden brown.
7. Repeat with the remaining batter, making about 12 pancakes total.
8. Serve the pancakes warm, topped with fresh berries.

Storage Instructions:
- Leftover pancakes can be stored in an airtight container in the refrigerator for up to 3 days.
- To reheat, place the pancakes on a baking sheet and warm in a 350°F oven for 5-10 minutes, or until heated through.

Tips:
- For extra fluffy pancakes, separate the egg and beat the egg white until stiff peaks form, then fold it into the batter.
- Adjust the amount of milk to achieve your desired pancake consistency.
- Feel free to use a combination of different fresh berries.

Nutrition Information:

Calories: 220 | Carbohydrates: 30g | Protein: 6g | Fat: 8g | Saturated Fat: 4g | Cholesterol: 55mg | Sodium: 370mg | Fiber: 2g | Sugar: 10g

PreparationTime: 10 minutes
Cook Time: 15 minutes
Total Time: 25 minutes
Serves: 4

Breakfast (23 Recipes)

2. Scrambled Eggs with Cheese

Ingredients:
- 2 eggs
- 2 tablespoons milk
- 1 tablespoon shredded cheddar cheese
- 1/2 teaspoon butter
- Salt and pepper to taste

PreparationTime: 5 minutes
Cook Time: 10 minutes
Total Time: 15 minutes
Serves: 1

Equipment:
- Small bowl
- Fork
- Non-stick skillet
- Spatula

Directions:
1. In a small bowl, whisk the eggs and milk together until well combined.

2. Heat a non-stick skillet over medium heat and melt the butter.

3. Pour the egg mixture into the skillet and let it sit for 30 seconds to 1 minute, until the edges start to set.

4. Using a spatula, gently push the eggs from the edge of the skillet towards the center, tilting the skillet to allow the uncooked egg to flow to the edges.

5. Continue this process, gently folding and stirring the eggs, until they are softly scrambled and no longer runny, about 2-3 minutes.

6. Remove the skillet from the heat and stir in the shredded cheddar cheese.

7. Season with salt and pepper to taste.

Storage Instructions:
- Scrambled eggs are best served immediately, as they can become dry and rubbery if reheated.

Tips:
- Use low-fat or non-fat milk to reduce the overall fat and calorie content.
- Add a small amount of chopped vegetables, such as spinach or tomatoes, for extra nutrition.
- Serve the scrambled eggs with whole-grain toast or a small side of fresh fruit for a balanced meal.

Nutrition Information:

Calories: 170 | Carbohydrates: 2g | Protein: 13g | Fat: 12g | Saturated Fat: 6g | Cholesterol: 260mg | Sodium: 320mg | Fiber: 0g | Sugar: 1g

Breakfast (23 Recipes)

3. Banana Oatmeal

Ingredients:
- 1/2 cup old-fashioned oats
- 1 cup milk (dairy, almond, or oat milk)
- 1 ripe banana, mashed
- 1 tablespoon honey (optional)
- 1/4 teaspoon ground cinnamon
- Pinch of salt

PreparationTime: 5 minutes
Cook Time: 10 minutes
Total Time: 15 minutes
Serves: 1

Equipment:
- Saucepan
- Spoon
- Bowl

Directions:

1. In a small saucepan, combine the oats and milk. Bring the mixture to a simmer over medium heat, stirring occasionally.

2. Once the oats have softened and the mixture has thickened, about 5-7 minutes, remove the saucepan from the heat.

3. Stir in the mashed banana, honey (if using), cinnamon, and a pinch of salt. Mix well until the banana is fully incorporated.

4. Transfer the banana oatmeal to a bowl and serve warm.

Storage Instructions:
- Leftover banana oatmeal can be stored in an airtight container in the refrigerator for up to 3 days.
- To reheat, simply add a splash of milk and microwave for 30-60 seconds, or until heated through.

Tips:
- For a creamier texture, use milk instead of water to cook the oats.
- Top the oatmeal with additional sliced banana, chopped nuts, or a drizzle of nut butter for extra flavor and nutrition.
- Adjust the amount of honey to your child's taste preference.
- Encourage your child to help mash the banana and mix the ingredients.

Nutrition Information:

Calories: 250 | Carbohydrates: 45g | Protein: 7g | Fat: 5g | Saturated Fat: 1g | Cholesterol: 5mg | Sodium: 105mg | Fiber: 5g | Sugar: 17g

Breakfast (23 Recipes)

4. Fruit Smoothie Bowl

Ingredients:
- 1 cup frozen mixed berries
(such as strawberries, blueberries, and raspberries)
- 1 banana, frozen
- 1/2 cup milk (dairy, almond, or oat milk)
- 1 tablespoon honey (optional)
- Toppings (such as sliced fresh fruit, granola, chia seeds, or shredded coconut)

PreparationTime: 10 minutes
Total Time: 10 minutes
Serves: 1

Equipment:
- Blender
- Bowl
- Spoon

Directions:
1. In a blender, combine the frozen mixed berries, frozen banana, and milk. Blend until smooth and creamy.

2. If desired, add the honey and blend again until well incorporated.

3. Pour the smoothie into a bowl.

4. Top the smoothie bowl with your choice of toppings, such as sliced fresh fruit, granola, chia seeds, or shredded coconut.

Storage Instructions:
- Enjoy the smoothie bowl immediately for the best texture and flavor.

- If you have any leftover smoothie, you can store it in an airtight container in the refrigerator for up to 2 days. Give it a quick blend before serving.

Tips:
- Use ripe, frozen bananas for a naturally sweet and creamy smoothie base.

- Adjust the amount of milk to achieve your desired consistency.

- Encourage your child to help choose and prepare the toppings.

- Offer a variety of toppings to make the smoothie bowl more visually appealing and fun to eat.

Nutrition Information:

Calories: 300 | Carbohydrates: 60g | Protein: 6g | Fat: 5g | Saturated Fat: 1g | Cholesterol: 5mg | Sodium: 55mg | Fiber: 9g | Sugar: 40g

Breakfast (23 Recipes)

5. Yogurt Parfait with Granola

Ingredients:
- 1 cup plain Greek yogurt
- 1/2 cup fresh berries
 (such as strawberries, blueberries, or raspberries)
- 1/4 cup granola

PreparationTime: 5 minutes
Total Time: 5 minutes
Serves: 1

Equipment:
- Glass or bowl
- Spoon

Directions:
1. In a glass or bowl, layer the yogurt, fresh berries, and granola, repeating the layers until you reach the top.

Storage Instructions:
- Enjoy the yogurt parfait immediately for the best texture and flavor.

- If you have any leftover parfait, you can store it in an airtight container in the refrigerator for up to 2 days.

Tips:
- Use your child's favorite fresh or frozen berries.

- Choose a granola that is low in added sugars and high in fiber and whole grains.

- Encourage your child to help assemble the parfait and choose the toppings.

- Offer a variety of toppings, such as sliced almonds, shredded coconut, or a drizzle of honey, to make the parfait more interesting.

Nutrition Information:

Calories: 220 | Carbohydrates: 30g | Protein: 15g | Fat: 5g | Saturated Fat: 2g | Cholesterol: 15mg | Sodium: 80mg | Fiber: 4g | Sugar: 18g

Breakfast (23 Recipes)

6. Avocado Toast

Ingredients:
- 1 slice whole-grain bread
- 1/2 ripe avocado, mashed
- 1 teaspoon lemon juice
- 1/4 teaspoon salt
- 1/8 teaspoon ground black pepper
- Optional toppings: cherry tomatoes, sliced cucumber, crumbled feta cheese, or a drizzle of olive oil

PreparationTime: 5 minutes
Cook Time: 2 minutes
Total Time: 7 minutes
Serves: 1

Equipment:
- Plate
- Fork or spoon
- Knife

Directions:

1. Toast the slice of whole-grain bread until lightly golden.

2. In a small bowl, mash the avocado with a fork or spoon. Stir in the lemon juice, salt, and black pepper until well combined.

3. Spread the mashed avocado mixture evenly over the toasted bread.

4. If desired, top the avocado toast with your choice of toppings, such as cherry tomatoes, sliced cucumber, crumbled feta cheese, or a drizzle of olive oil.

Storage Instructions:

- Avocado toast is best enjoyed immediately, as the avocado can brown and the bread can become soggy if stored.

Tips:
- Use ripe, creamy avocados for the best flavor and texture.
- Encourage your child to help mash the avocado and assemble the toast.
- Offer a variety of toppings to make the avocado toast more appealing and nutritious.
- Serve the avocado toast with a small side of fresh fruit or a glass of milk for a balanced meal.

Nutrition Information:

Calories: 250 | Carbohydrates: 30g | Protein: 7g | Fat: 13g | Saturated Fat: 2g | Cholesterol: 0mg | Sodium: 450mg | Fiber: 9g | Sugar: 3g

Breakfast (23 Recipes)

7. Blueberry Muffins

Ingredients:
- 2 cups all-purpose flour
- 1 tablespoon baking powder
- 1/2 teaspoon salt
- 1/2 cup unsalted butter, melted and slightly cooled
- 3/4 cup granulated sugar
- 1 egg
- 1 cup milk
- 1 teaspoon vanilla extract
- 1 cup fresh or frozen blueberries

PreparationTime: 15 minutes
Cook Time: 20 minutes
Total Time: 35 minutes
Serves: 12 muffins

Equipment:
- Muffin tin
- Mixing bowl
- Whisk
- Spoon
- Oven

Directions:
1. Preheat the oven to 400°F (200°C). Grease a 12-cup muffin tin or line it with paper liners.
2. In a large mixing bowl, whisk together the flour, baking powder, and salt.
3. In a separate bowl, whisk together the melted butter, sugar, egg, milk, and vanilla extract.
4. Gently fold the wet ingredients into the dry ingredients, being careful not to overmix. Fold in the blueberries.
5. Divide the batter evenly among the prepared muffin cups, filling them about 3/4 full.
6. Bake for 18-20 minutes, or until a toothpick inserted into the center comes out clean.
7. Allow the muffins to cool in the tin for 5 minutes before transferring them to a wire rack to cool completely.

Storage Instructions:
- Store the cooled muffins in an airtight container at room temperature for up to 3 days.
- You can also freeze the muffins for up to 3 months. Thaw at room temperature before serving.

Tips:
- Use fresh or frozen blueberries for the best flavor and texture.
- Encourage your child to help measure the ingredients and mix the batter.
- Serve the muffins warm, with a glass of milk or a piece of fruit, for a delicious and nutritious snack.

Nutrition Information:

Calories: 200 | Carbohydrates: 30g | Protein: 3g | Fat: 8g | Saturated Fat: 5g | Cholesterol: 35mg | Sodium: 210mg | Fiber: 1g | Sugar: 15g

Breakfast (23 Recipes)

8. French Toast with Maple Syrup

Ingredients:
- 4 eggs
- 1/2 cup milk
- 1 teaspoon vanilla extract
- 1/4 teaspoon ground cinnamon
- Pinch of salt
- 8 slices of whole-grain bread
- 2 tablespoons unsalted butter
- 1/4 cup pure maple syrup

PreparationTime: 10 minutes
Cook Time: 15 minutes
Total Time: 25 minutes
Serves: 4

Equipment:
- Shallow bowl
- Whisk
- Skillet or griddle
- Spatula

Directions:
1. In a shallow bowl, whisk together the eggs, milk, vanilla extract, cinnamon, and salt until well combined.

2. Dip the bread slices into the egg mixture, coating both sides evenly.

3. Melt the butter in a skillet or on a griddle over medium heat.

4. Cook the dipped bread slices for 2-3 minutes per side, or until golden brown.

5. Serve the French toast warm, drizzled with the maple syrup.

Storage Instructions:
- Leftover French toast can be stored in an airtight container in the refrigerator for up to 3 days.
- To reheat, place the French toast slices on a baking sheet and warm in a 350°F oven for 5-10 minutes, or until heated through.

Tips:
- Use day-old or slightly stale bread for the best texture.
- Encourage your child to help dip the bread slices in the egg mixture.
- Offer additional toppings, such as fresh berries, whipped cream, or a dusting of powdered sugar, to make the French toast more appealing.
- Serve the French toast with a side of fresh fruit or a glass of milk for a balanced meal.

Nutrition Information:

Calories: 280 | Carbohydrates: 35g | Protein: 10g | Fat: 11g | Saturated Fat: 5g | Cholesterol: 185mg | Sodium: 320mg | Fiber: 3g | Sugar: 12g

Breakfast (23 Recipes)

9. Breakfast Burrito

Ingredients:
- 1 whole-wheat tortilla
- 2 eggs, scrambled
- 2 tablespoons shredded cheddar cheese
- 2 tablespoons diced bell pepper
- 2 tablespoons diced onion
- 1 tablespoon salsa (optional)
- Salt and pepper to taste

Equipment:
- Skillet
- Mixing bowl
- Spatula
- Plate

PreparationTime: 10 minutes
Cook Time: 15 minutes
Total Time: 25 minutes
Serves: 1

Directions:
1. In a skillet over medium heat, sauté the diced bell pepper and onion until softened, about 3-5 minutes.
2. In a mixing bowl, whisk the eggs and season with a pinch of salt and pepper.
3. Pour the egg mixture into the skillet with the vegetables and scramble the eggs until cooked through, about 2-3 minutes.
4. Remove the skillet from heat and stir in the shredded cheddar cheese.
5. Warm the whole-wheat tortilla according to package instructions.
6. Place the scrambled egg mixture onto the center of the tortilla.
7. Fold the bottom of the tortilla up, then fold in the sides and roll up tightly to create a burrito.
8. Serve the breakfast burrito warm, with a side of salsa if desired.

Storage Instructions:
- Leftover breakfast burritos can be wrapped in foil or parchment paper and stored in the refrigerator for up to 3 days.
- To reheat, remove the foil or parchment paper and microwave the burrito for 1-2 minutes, or until heated through.

Tips:
- Encourage your child to help prepare the fillings and assemble the burrito.
- Customize the fillings to your child's preferences, such as adding diced ham, spinach, or mushrooms.
- Serve the breakfast burrito with a side of fresh fruit or a small glass of milk for a balanced meal.

Nutrition Information:

Calories: 320 | Carbohydrates: 30g | Protein: 18g | Fat: 15g | Saturated Fat: 7g | Cholesterol: 215mg | Sodium: 550mg | Fiber: 5g | Sugar: 4g

Breakfast (23 Recipes)

10. Chocolate Chip Waffles

Ingredients:
- 1 1/2 cups all-purpose flour
- 1 tablespoon baking powder
- 1 tablespoon granulated sugar
- 1/4 teaspoon salt
- 1 1/4 cups milk
- 1/3 cup unsalted butter, melted
- 1 egg
- 1 teaspoon vanilla extract
- 1/2 cup semi-sweet chocolate chips

PreparationTime: 10 minutes
Cook Time: 15 minutes
Total Time: 25 minutes
Serves: 4 (8 waffles)

Equipment:
- Waffle iron
- Mixing bowl
- Whisk
- Ladle or measuring cup

Directions:
1. In a large mixing bowl, whisk together the flour, baking powder, sugar, and salt.
2. In a separate bowl, whisk together the milk, melted butter, egg, and vanilla extract.
3. Pour the wet ingredients into the dry ingredients and whisk until just combined (do not overmix).
4. Gently fold in the chocolate chips.
5. Preheat your waffle iron and lightly grease it if necessary.
6. Scoop the batter onto the hot waffle iron, using about 1/2 cup of batter per waffle. Cook for 3-5 minutes, or until the waffles are golden brown and crispy.
7. Serve the chocolate chip waffles warm, with your child's favorite toppings, such as maple syrup, whipped cream, or fresh berries.

Storage Instructions:
- Leftover waffles can be stored in an airtight container in the refrigerator for up to 3 days.
- To reheat, place the waffles in a toaster or oven at 350°F (175°C) for 2-3 minutes, or until heated through.

Tips:
- Encourage your child to help measure the ingredients and fold in the chocolate chips.
- Experiment with different mix-ins, such as chopped nuts, shredded coconut, or a sprinkle of cinnamon.
- Serve the waffles with a side of fresh fruit or a glass of milk for a balanced breakfast.

Nutrition Information:

Calories: 290 | Carbohydrates: 37g | Protein: 7g | Fat: 14g | Saturated Fat: 8g | Cholesterol: 55mg | Sodium: 390mg | Fiber: 2g | Sugar: 12g

Breakfast (23 Recipes)

11. Cinnamon Raisin Bagels

Ingredients:
- 3 cups (375g) bread flour
- 1 teaspoon salt
- 1 teaspoon ground cinnamon
- 1 tablespoon granulated sugar
- 1 teaspoon active dry yeast
- 1 1/4 cups (295ml) warm water
- 1 cup (150g) raisins

Equipment:
- Large mixing bowl
- Wooden spoon
- Dough hook (for a stand mixer)
- Baking sheet
- Parchment paper
- Slotted spoon
- Oven

PreparationTime: 20 minutes
Proofing Time: 1 hour
Cook Time: 20 minutes
Total Time: 1 hour 40 minutes
Serves: 8 bagels

Nutrition Information:
Calories: 240 | Carbohydrates: 48g | Protein: 7g | Fat: 2g | Saturated Fat: 0g | Cholesterol: 0mg | Sodium: 380mg | Fiber: 3g | Sugar: 7g

Directions:
1. In a large mixing bowl, combine the bread flour, salt, cinnamon, sugar, and yeast. Stir to mix.
2. Add the warm water and use a wooden spoon to mix until a shaggy dough forms.
3. Turn the dough out onto a lightly floured surface and knead for about 10 minutes, until the dough becomes smooth and elastic.
4. Place the dough in a lightly greased bowl, cover, and let it rise for 1 hour, or until doubled in size.
5. Punch down the dough to release any air bubbles. Knead in the raisins until evenly distributed.
6. Divide the dough into 8 equal pieces. Roll each piece into a ball, then use your fingers to poke a hole in the center and gently stretch the dough to form a bagel shape.
7. Bring a large pot of water to a boil. Carefully drop the bagels into the boiling water, a few at a time, and cook for 1 minute per side.
8. Remove the boiled bagels with a slotted spoon and place them on a parchment-lined baking sheet.
9. Bake the bagels at 400°F (200°C) for 20 minutes, or until golden brown.
10. Allow the bagels to cool on a wire rack before serving.

Storage Instructions:
- Leftover bagels can be stored in an airtight container at room temperature for up to 5 days.
- To freeze, wrap the bagels individually in plastic wrap or foil and store in a freezer-safe bag for up to 3 months.

Tips:
- Encourage your child to help shape the bagels and add the raisins.
- Serve the cinnamon raisin bagels with cream cheese, nut butter, or your child's favorite toppings.
- For a fun twist, try adding other dried fruits or nuts to the dough.

Breakfast (23 Recipes)

12. Spinach and Cheese Omelet

Ingredients:
- 2 eggs
- 1 tablespoon milk
- 1 tablespoon shredded cheddar cheese
- 1/4 cup fresh spinach, chopped
- 1/2 teaspoon butter
- Salt and pepper to taste

PreparationTime: 5 minutes
Cook Time: 10 minutes
Total Time: 15 minutes
Serves: 1

Equipment:
- Small bowl
- Fork
- Non-stick skillet
- Spatula

Directions:
1. In a small bowl, whisk the eggs and milk together until well combined.
2. Heat a non-stick skillet over medium heat and melt the butter.
3. Pour the egg mixture into the skillet and let it sit for 30 seconds to 1 minute, until the edges start to set.
4. Using a spatula, gently push the eggs from the edge of the skillet towards the center, tilting the skillet to allow the uncooked egg to flow to the edges.
5. Continue this process, gently folding and stirring the eggs, until they are softly scrambled and no longer runny, about 2-3 minutes.
6. Sprinkle the chopped spinach and shredded cheddar cheese over the eggs.
7. Fold the omelet in half and slide it onto a plate.
8. Season with salt and pepper to taste.

Storage Instructions:
- Omelets are best served immediately, as they can become dry and rubbery if reheated.

Tips:
- Use fresh, high-quality ingredients for the best flavor and texture.
- Encourage your child to help prepare the ingredients and assemble the omelet.
- Serve the omelet with a slice of whole-grain toast or a small side of fresh fruit for a balanced meal.
- Experiment with different fillings, such as diced tomatoes, mushrooms, or bell peppers, to keep the omelet interesting.

Nutrition Information:

Calories: 190 | Carbohydrates: 3g | Protein: 14g | Fat: 13g | Saturated Fat: 6g | Cholesterol: 260mg | Sodium: 320mg | Fiber: 1g | Sugar: 1g

Breakfast (23 Recipes)

13. Apple Cinnamon Porridge

Ingredients:
- 1/2 cup rolled oats
- 1 cup milk (dairy, almond, or oat milk)
- 1/2 apple, peeled, cored, and diced
- 1 teaspoon ground cinnamon
- 1 tablespoon honey (optional)
- Pinch of salt

PreparationTime: 5 minutes
Cook Time: 15 minutes
Total Time: 20 minutes
Serves: 1

Equipment:
- Saucepan
- Spoon
- Bowl

Directions:

1. In a small saucepan, combine the rolled oats and milk. Bring the mixture to a simmer over medium heat, stirring occasionally.

2. Once the oats have softened and the porridge has thickened, about 10-12 minutes, stir in the diced apple, cinnamon, honey (if using), and a pinch of salt.

3. Continue cooking for an additional 2-3 minutes, or until the apple pieces are tender.

4. Remove the saucepan from the heat and transfer the apple cinnamon porridge to a bowl.

Storage Instructions:
- Leftover porridge can be stored in an airtight container in the refrigerator for up to 3 days.
- To reheat, add a splash of milk and microwave for 30-60 seconds, or until heated through.

Tips:
- Use a crisp, tart apple variety, such as Granny Smith or Honeycrisp, for the best flavor.
- Adjust the amount of honey to your child's taste preference.
- Top the porridge with additional sliced apples, a sprinkle of chopped nuts, or a drizzle of nut butter for extra flavor and nutrition.
- Encourage your child to help prepare the ingredients and stir the porridge as it cooks.

Nutrition Information:

Calories: 250 | Carbohydrates: 45g | Protein: 7g | Fat: 5g | Saturated Fat: 1g | Cholesterol: 5mg | Sodium: 105mg | Fiber: 6g | Sugar: 17g

14. Peanut Butter Banana Sandwich

Ingredients:
- 2 slices of whole-grain bread
- 2 tablespoons creamy peanut butter
- 1 ripe banana, sliced

Equipment:
- Knife
- Plate

Directions:

1. Spread the peanut butter evenly on one slice of bread.

2. Arrange the sliced banana on top of the peanut butter.

3. Place the second slice of bread on top to create a sandwich.

Storage Instructions:
- Peanut butter and banana sandwiches are best enjoyed immediately, as the banana can become brown and the bread can become soggy if stored.

Tips:
- Use ripe, sweet bananas for the best flavor.

- Encourage your child to help prepare the sandwich by spreading the peanut butter and arranging the banana slices.

- For a variation, try using almond butter or cashew butter instead of peanut butter.

- Serve the sandwich with a small side of fresh fruit or a glass of milk for a balanced snack.

Nutrition Information:

Calories: 320 | Carbohydrates: 40g | Protein: 12g | Fat: 15g | Saturated Fat: 2g | Cholesterol: 0mg | Sodium: 320mg | Fiber: 6g | Sugar: 12g

PreparationTime: 5 minutes
Total Time: 5 minutes
Serves: 1

Breakfast (23 Recipes)

15. Mini Quiches

Ingredients:
- 1 sheet of refrigerated pie crust
- 6 eggs
- 1/2 cup milk
- 1/4 teaspoon salt
- 1/8 teaspoon black pepper
- 1/2 cup shredded cheddar cheese
- 1/4 cup diced ham or cooked bacon (optional)
- 2 tablespoons diced bell pepper (optional)

PreparationTime: 15 minutes
Cook Time: 20 minutes
Total Time: 35 minutes
Serves: 12 mini quiches

Equipment:
- Muffin tin
- Mixing bowl
- Whisk
- Spoon
- Oven

Directions:
1. Preheat the oven to 375°F (190°C). Grease a 12-cup muffin tin.
2. Unroll the pie crust and use a 3-inch round cookie cutter to cut out 12 circles.
3. Gently press the pie crust circles into the prepared muffin cups, pressing them into the sides and bottom.
4. In a mixing bowl, whisk together the eggs, milk, salt, and black pepper until well combined.
5. Divide the egg mixture evenly among the muffin cups, filling them about 3/4 full.
6. Sprinkle the shredded cheddar cheese and any desired toppings (ham, bacon, or bell pepper) over the egg mixture.
7. Bake for 18-20 minutes, or until the quiches are set and the crust is golden brown.
8. Allow the mini quiches to cool in the muffin tin for 5 minutes before removing them.

Storage Instructions:
- Cooled mini quiches can be stored in an airtight container in the refrigerator for up to 3 days.
- To reheat, place the quiches on a baking sheet and warm in a 350°F (175°C) oven for 5-7 minutes, or until heated through.

Tips:
- Encourage your child to help prepare the ingredients and assemble the mini quiches.
- Experiment with different fillings, such as spinach, mushrooms, or diced tomatoes, to keep the quiches interesting.
- Serve the mini quiches with a side of fresh fruit or a small salad for a balanced meal.

Nutrition Information:

Calories: 150 | Carbohydrates: 10g | Protein: 8g | Fat: 9g | Saturated Fat: 4g | Cholesterol: 105mg | Sodium: 300mg | Fiber: 1g | Sugar: 2g

Breakfast (23 Recipes)

16. Breakfast Quesadillas

Ingredients:
- 4 whole-wheat tortillas
- 4 eggs, scrambled
- 1/2 cup shredded cheddar cheese
- 2 tablespoons diced bell pepper
- 2 tablespoons diced onion
- Salt and pepper to taste
- Butter or oil for cooking

Equipment:
- Skillet
- Spatula
- Plate

PreparationTime: 10 minutes
Cook Time: 10 minutes
Total Time: 20 minutes
Serves: 2 quesadillas (4 halves)

Nutrition Information:
Calories: 380 | Carbohydrates: 35g | Protein: 20g | Fat: 18g | Saturated Fat: 8g | Cholesterol: 215mg | Sodium: 680mg | Fiber: 5g | Sugar: 3g

Directions:
1. In a skillet over medium heat, sauté the diced bell pepper and onion until softened, about 3-5 minutes.
2. In a separate bowl, scramble the eggs and season with a pinch of salt and pepper.
3. Add the scrambled eggs to the skillet with the vegetables and cook, stirring occasionally, until the eggs are fully cooked, about 2-3 minutes.
4. Remove the egg mixture from the heat and set aside.
5. Wipe the skillet clean and place it back over medium heat. Add a small amount of butter or oil to the pan.
6. Place one tortilla in the skillet and top it with half of the scrambled egg mixture and half of the shredded cheddar cheese.
7. Place a second tortilla on top to create a quesadilla.
8. Cook the quesadilla for 2-3 minutes per side, or until the tortilla is golden brown and the cheese is melted.
9. Repeat steps 6-8 to make a second quesadilla.
10. Cut each quesadilla in half and serve warm.

Storage Instructions:
- Leftover breakfast quesadillas can be wrapped in foil or parchment paper and stored in the refrigerator for up to 3 days.
- To reheat, remove the foil or parchment paper and microwave the quesadilla for 1-2 minutes, or until heated through.

Tips:
- Encourage your child to help prepare the fillings and assemble the quesadillas.
- Customize the fillings to your child's preferences, such as adding diced ham, spinach, or mushrooms.
- Serve the breakfast quesadillas with a side of salsa, guacamole, or a small fruit salad for a balanced meal.

Breakfast (23 Recipes)

17. Berry Breakfast Bars

Ingredients:
- 1 1/2 cups old-fashioned oats
- 1 cup whole-wheat flour
- 1/2 cup brown sugar
- 1 teaspoon baking powder
- 1/4 teaspoon salt
- 1/2 cup unsalted butter, melted
- 1 egg
- 1 teaspoon vanilla extract
- 1 cup mixed berries (such as blueberries, raspberries, and blackberries)

Equipment:
- 8x8-inch baking pan
- Mixing bowl
- Spoon
- Oven

PreparationTime: 15 minutes
Cook Time: 25 minutes
Total Time: 40 minutes
Serves: 9 bars

Directions:
1. Preheat the oven to 350°F (175°C). Grease an 8x8-inch baking pan.
2. In a large mixing bowl, combine the oats, whole-wheat flour, brown sugar, baking powder, and salt. Stir to mix.
3. Add the melted butter, egg, and vanilla extract to the dry ingredients. Stir until just combined.
4. Gently fold in the mixed berries.
5. Press the mixture evenly into the prepared baking pan.
6. Bake for 25-30 minutes, or until the edges are golden brown and the center is set.
7. Allow the bars to cool completely in the pan before cutting into 9 squares.

Storage Instructions:
- Store the cooled breakfast bars in an airtight container at room temperature for up to 5 days.
- You can also freeze the bars for up to 3 months. Thaw at room temperature before serving.

Tips:
- Use a combination of your child's favorite berries for the best flavor.
- Encourage your child to help measure the ingredients and mix the batter.
- Serve the breakfast bars with a glass of milk or a piece of fresh fruit for a balanced snack.
- For a crunchier texture, sprinkle the top of the batter with chopped nuts or a streusel topping before baking.

Nutrition Information:

Calories: 220 | Carbohydrates: 32g | Protein: 4g | Fat: 9g | Saturated Fat: 5g | Cholesterol: 35mg | Sodium: 120mg | Fiber: 3g | Sugar: 15g

Breakfast (23 Recipes)

18. Ham and Cheese Croissant

Ingredients:
- 1 croissant, sliced in half horizontally
- 2 slices of ham
- 2 slices of cheddar cheese
- 1 teaspoon butter

Equipment:
- Baking sheet
- Oven or toaster oven

PreparationTime: 5 minutes
Cook Time: 10 minutes
Total Time: 15 minutes
Serves: 1

Directions:

1. Preheat the oven or toaster oven to 350°F (175°C).

2. Place the croissant halves on a baking sheet.

3. Layer the ham and cheddar cheese slices on the bottom half of the croissant.

4. Place the top half of the croissant back on top.

5. Spread the butter evenly over the top of the croissant.

6. Bake for 8-10 minutes, or until the cheese is melted and the croissant is lightly golden.

7. Remove the ham and cheese croissant from the oven and let it cool for a minute before serving.

Storage Instructions:
- Leftover ham and cheese croissants can be stored in an airtight container in the refrigerator for up to 3 days.
- To reheat, place the croissant on a baking sheet and warm in a 350°F (175°C) oven for 5-7 minutes, or until heated through.

Tips:
- Use high-quality, thinly sliced ham and cheddar cheese for the best flavor.
- Encourage your child to help assemble the croissant.
- Serve the ham and cheese croissant with a side of fresh fruit or a small salad for a balanced meal.
- For a variation, try adding a thin slice of tomato or a few spinach leaves to the croissant.

Nutrition Information:

Calories: 350 | Carbohydrates: 30g | Protein: 15g | Fat: 19g | Saturated Fat: 10g | Cholesterol: 55mg | Sodium: 900mg | Fiber: 2g | Sugar: 3g

Breakfast (23 Recipes)

19. Mango Chia Pudding

Ingredients:
- 1 cup unsweetened almond milk
- 3 tablespoons chia seeds
- 1 ripe mango, peeled and diced
- 1 tablespoon honey (optional)
- 1/4 teaspoon vanilla extract

PreparationTime: 10 minutes
Chilling Time: 2 hours
Total Time: 2 hours 10 minutes
Serves: 2

Equipment:
- Mason jar or small bowl with lid
- Spoon
- Refrigerator

Directions:

1. In a mason jar or small bowl with a lid, combine the almond milk and chia seeds. Stir well.

2. Cover the jar or bowl and refrigerate for at least 2 hours, or up to 24 hours, stirring occasionally, until the chia seeds have thickened the mixture into a pudding-like consistency.

3. Once the chia pudding has set, stir in the diced mango, honey (if using), and vanilla extract until well combined.

4. Serve chilled, or refrigerate for up to 3 days.

Storage Instructions:
- The mango chia pudding can be stored in an airtight container in the refrigerator for up to 3 days.

Tips:
- Use ripe, sweet mangoes for the best flavor.

- Adjust the amount of honey to your child's taste preference.

- Top the chia pudding with additional diced mango, toasted coconut flakes, or a sprinkle of cinnamon for extra flavor and texture.

- Encourage your child to help prepare the ingredients and assemble the chia pudding.

Nutrition Information:

Calories: 200 | Carbohydrates: 30g | Protein: 5g | Fat: 8g | Saturated Fat: 1g | Cholesterol: 0mg | Sodium: 75mg | Fiber: 7g | Sugar: 20g

Breakfast (23 Recipes)

20. Egg Muffins with Veggies

Ingredients:
- 6 eggs
- 1/4 cup diced bell pepper
- 1/4 cup diced onion
- 1/4 cup diced spinach
- 2 tablespoons shredded cheddar cheese
- Salt and pepper to taste

Equipment:
- Muffin tin
- Mixing bowl
- Whisk
- Spoon
- Oven

PreparationTime: 10 minutes
Cook Time: 20 minutes
Total Time: 30 minutes
Serves: 6 muffins

Directions:

1. Preheat the oven to 350°F (175°C). Grease a 6-cup muffin tin.

2. In a mixing bowl, whisk the eggs together until well combined.

3. Stir in the diced bell pepper, onion, and spinach.

4. Season the egg mixture with a pinch of salt and pepper.

5. Divide the egg mixture evenly among the prepared muffin cups, filling them about 3/4 full.

6. Sprinkle the shredded cheddar cheese on top of each muffin.

7. Bake for 18-20 minutes, or until the egg muffins are set and the cheese is melted.

8. Allow the muffins to cool in the tin for 5 minutes before removing them.

Storage Instructions:
- Cooled egg muffins can be stored in an airtight container in the refrigerator for up to 4 days.
- To reheat, place the muffins on a baking sheet and warm in a 350°F (175°C) oven for 5-7 minutes, or until heated through.

Tips:
- Encourage your child to help prepare the vegetables and assemble the muffins.
- Experiment with different vegetable combinations, such as diced tomatoes, mushrooms, or broccoli.
- Serve the egg muffins with a side of fresh fruit or a small yogurt for a balanced breakfast or snack.

Nutrition Information:

Calories: 110 | Carbohydrates: 3g | Protein: 9g | Fat: 7g | Saturated Fat: 3g | Cholesterol: 185mg | Sodium: 180mg | Fiber: 1g | Sugar: 2g

Breakfast (23 Recipes)

21. Breakfast Tacos

Ingredients:
- 4 small corn or flour tortillas
- 4 eggs, scrambled
- 1/4 cup diced bell pepper
- 1/4 cup diced onion
- 2 tablespoons shredded cheddar cheese
- 2 tablespoons salsa (optional)
- Salt and pepper to taste

PreparationTime: 10 minutes
Cook Time: 15 minutes
Total Time: 25 minutes
Serves: 4 tacos

Equipment:
- Skillet
- Mixing bowl
- Whisk
- Spoon

Directions:
1. In a skillet over medium heat, sauté the diced bell pepper and onion until softened, about 3-5 minutes.
2. In a mixing bowl, whisk the eggs together until well combined. Season with a pinch of salt and pepper.
3. Pour the egg mixture into the skillet with the vegetables and scramble the eggs until cooked through, about 2-3 minutes.
4. Remove the skillet from the heat and stir in the shredded cheddar cheese.
5. Warm the tortillas according to package instructions.
6. Divide the scrambled egg mixture evenly among the tortillas.
7. Top each taco with a spoonful of salsa, if desired.

Storage Instructions:
- Leftover breakfast tacos can be stored in an airtight container in the refrigerator for up to 3 days.
- To reheat, place the tacos on a baking sheet and warm in a 350°F (175°C) oven for 5-7 minutes, or until heated through.

Tips:
- Encourage your child to help prepare the vegetables and assemble the tacos.
- Customize the fillings to your child's preferences, such as adding diced avocado, crumbled bacon, or diced tomatoes.
- Serve the breakfast tacos with a side of fresh fruit or a small glass of milk for a balanced meal.

Nutrition Information:

Calories: 220 | Carbohydrates: 20g | Protein: 13g | Fat: 11g | Saturated Fat: 5g | Cholesterol: 215mg | Sodium: 420mg | Fiber: 3g | Sugar: 3g

Breakfast (23 Recipes)

22. Pumpkin Spice Pancakes

Ingredients:
- 1 1/4 cups all-purpose flour
- 2 tablespoons brown sugar
- 2 teaspoons baking powder
- 1 teaspoon ground cinnamon
- 1/2 teaspoon ground ginger
- 1/4 teaspoon ground nutmeg
- 1/4 teaspoon salt
- 1 cup milk
- 1/2 cup canned pumpkin puree
- 1 egg
- 2 tablespoons unsalted butter, melted
- 1 teaspoon vanilla extract

Equipment:
- Mixing bowl
- Whisk
- Griddle or non-stick skillet
- Spatula

PreparationTime: 10 minutes
Cook Time: 15 minutes
Total Time: 25 minutes
Serves: 4 (8 pancakes)

Nutrition Information:
Calories: 230 |
Carbohydrates: 34g | Protein:
6g | Fat: 8g | Saturated Fat:
4g | Cholesterol: 55mg |
Sodium: 370mg | Fiber: 2g |
Sugar: 10g

Directions:
1. In a large mixing bowl, whisk together the flour, brown sugar, baking powder, cinnamon, ginger, nutmeg, and salt.
2. In a separate bowl, whisk together the milk, pumpkin puree, egg, melted butter, and vanilla extract.
3. Pour the wet ingredients into the dry ingredients and whisk until just combined (do not overmix).
4. Heat a griddle or non-stick skillet over medium heat. Lightly grease the surface.
5. Scoop about 1/4 cup of batter onto the hot surface and cook for 2-3 minutes, or until bubbles start to form on the surface.
6. Flip the pancake and cook for an additional 1-2 minutes, or until golden brown.
7. Repeat with the remaining batter, making about 16 pancakes total.
8. Serve the pumpkin spice pancakes warm, with your child's favorite toppings, such as maple syrup, whipped cream, or a dusting of powdered sugar.

Storage Instructions:
- Leftover pancakes can be stored in an airtight container in the refrigerator for up to 3 days.
- To reheat, place the pancakes on a baking sheet and warm in a 350°F (175°C) oven for 5-10 minutes, or until heated through.

Tips:
- Encourage your child to help measure the ingredients and mix the batter.
- Adjust the amount of milk to achieve your desired pancake consistency.
- Serve the pancakes with a side of fresh fruit or a glass of milk for a balanced breakfast.

Breakfast (23 Recipes)

23. Strawberry Smoothie

Ingredients:
- 1 cup frozen strawberries
- 1 banana, frozen
- 1/2 cup milk (dairy, almond, or oat milk)
- 1 tablespoon honey (optional)

PreparationTime: 5 minutes
Total Time: 5 minutes
Serves: 1

Equipment:
- Blender

Directions:
1. In a blender, combine the frozen strawberries, frozen banana, and milk.

2. If desired, add the honey and blend until smooth and creamy.

Storage Instructions:
- Enjoy the strawberry smoothie immediately for the best texture and flavor.

- If you have any leftover smoothie, you can store it in an airtight container in the refrigerator for up to 2 days. Give it a quick blend before serving.

Tips:
- Use ripe, frozen bananas for a naturally sweet and creamy smoothie base.

- Adjust the amount of milk to achieve your desired consistency.

- Encourage your child to help measure the ingredients and blend the smoothie.

- For extra nutrition, add a handful of spinach or a tablespoon of nut butter.

Nutrition Information:

Calories: 220 | Carbohydrates: 45g | Protein: 5g | Fat: 3g | Saturated Fat: 0g | Cholesterol: 0mg | Sodium: 45mg | Fiber: 6g | Sugar: 30g

24. Apple Slices with Peanut Butter

Ingredients:
- 1 medium apple, cored and sliced
- 2 tablespoons creamy peanut butter

Equipment:
- Knife
- Plate

PreparationTime: 5 minutes
Total Time: 5 minutes
Serves: 1

Directions:
1. Wash and slice the apple, removing the core.

2. Arrange the apple slices on a plate.

3. Serve the apple slices with the peanut butter on the side for dipping.

Storage Instructions:

- Leftover apple slices can be stored in an airtight container in the refrigerator for up to 3 days.
- The peanut butter can be stored at room temperature.

Tips:
- Use a crisp, tart apple variety, such as Granny Smith or Honeycrisp, for the best flavor.
- Encourage your child to help prepare the apple slices.
- For a variation, try using almond butter or cashew butter instead of peanut butter.
- Serve the apple slices and peanut butter with a small glass of milk for a balanced snack.

Nutrition Information:

Calories: 180 | Carbohydrates: 20g | Protein: 5g | Fat: 10g | Saturated Fat: 1.5g | Cholesterol: 0mg | Sodium: 105mg | Fiber: 4g | Sugar: 15g

25. Carrot and Cucumber Sticks with Hummus

Ingredients:
- 1 medium carrot, peeled and cut into sticks
- 1 small cucumber, cut into sticks
- 2 tablespoons hummus

Equipment:
- Knife
- Cutting board
- Small bowl

Directions:
1. Wash and peel the carrot. Cut it into thin, stick-shaped pieces.

2. Wash the cucumber and cut it into thin, stick-shaped pieces.

3. Arrange the carrot and cucumber sticks on a plate or in a small bowl.

4. Serve the vegetable sticks with the hummus on the side for dipping.

Storage Instructions:
- Leftover carrot and cucumber sticks can be stored in an airtight container in the refrigerator for up to 3 days.
- The hummus can be stored in an airtight container in the refrigerator for up to 1 week.

Tips:
- Encourage your child to help prepare the vegetables by washing, peeling, and cutting them.
- Try different types of hummus, such as roasted red pepper or garlic, to keep the snack interesting.
- Serve the carrot and cucumber sticks with hummus as a healthy, balanced snack.
- For a variation, try pairing the vegetable sticks with a low-fat ranch dressing or Greek yogurt-based dip.

Nutrition Information:

Calories: 80 | Carbohydrates: 10g | Protein: 3g | Fat: 4g | Saturated Fat: 0.5g | Cholesterol: 0mg | Sodium: 160mg | Fiber: 3g | Sugar: 5g

PreparationTime: 10 minutes
Total Time: 10 minutes
Serves: 1

Snacks (23 Recipes)

26. Cheese and Crackers

Ingredients:
- 4-5 whole grain crackers
- 1 ounce cheddar or mozzarella cheese, cut into slices or cubes
- 1 tablespoon grapes or apple slices (optional)

Equipment:
- Cutting board
- Knife
- Plate

PreparationTime: 5 minutes
Cook Time: 0 minutes
Total Time: 5 minutes
Serves: 1

Directions:

1. Arrange the crackers on a plate.

2. Place the cheese slices or cubes on top of the crackers.

3. If desired, add the grapes or apple slices alongside the crackers and cheese.

Storage Instructions:
- This snack is best served immediately, but any leftovers can be stored in an airtight container in the refrigerator for up to 2 days.

Tips:
- Choose whole grain crackers for added fiber and nutrients.

- Vary the type of cheese to keep it interesting, such as cheddar, mozzarella, or gouda.

- Add a small amount of fruit for a touch of sweetness and extra nutrition.

- Encourage the 9-year-old to help assemble the snack for a fun, interactive experience.

Nutrition Information:
Calories: 150 | Total Fat: 7g | Saturated Fat: 4g | Cholesterol: 20mg | Sodium: 250mg | Total Carbohydrates: 15g | Dietary Fiber: 2g | Total Sugars: 2g | Protein: 7g

Snacks (23 Recipes)

27. Homemade Trail Mix

Ingredients:
- 1/2 cup roasted unsalted almonds
- 1/2 cup roasted unsalted cashews
- 1/2 cup dried cranberries
- 1/4 cup mini chocolate chips
- 1/4 cup roasted unsalted pumpkin seeds
- 1/4 cup roasted unsalted sunflower seeds

PreparationTime: 10 minutes
Cook Time: 0 minutes
Total Time: 10 minutes
Serves: 4

Equipment:
- Mixing bowl
- Measuring cups

Directions:

1. In a large mixing bowl, combine the almonds, cashews, dried cranberries, chocolate chips, pumpkin seeds, and sunflower seeds.

2. Stir the ingredients together until well mixed.

Storage Instructions:
- Store the trail mix in an airtight container at room temperature for up to 2 weeks.

Tips:
- Adjust the ingredient amounts to suit the 9-year-old's preferences. You can add or remove items based on their likes and dislikes.

- Consider using a variety of dried fruits, such as raisins, apricots, or mango, for added sweetness and texture.

- Encourage the 9-year-old to help assemble the trail mix for a fun, hands-on activity.

- Portion the trail mix into individual servings for easy snacking.

Nutrition Information:
Calories: 200 | Total Fat: 14g | Saturated Fat: 3g | Cholesterol: 0mg | Sodium: 50mg | Total Carbohydrates: 16g | Dietary Fiber: 3g | Total Sugars: 10g | Protein: 6g

Snacks (23 Recipes)

28. Fruit Kabobs

Ingredients:
- 1 cup cubed watermelon
- 1 cup cubed pineapple
- 1 cup grapes
- 1 cup cubed cantaloupe
- 1 cup strawberries, halved

PreparationTime: 15 minutes
Cook Time: 0 minutes
Total Time: 15 minutes
Serves: 4

Equipment:
- Cutting board
- Knife
- Skewers

Directions:
1. Wash and prepare the fruit:

   - Cube the watermelon and cantaloupe.

   - Cut the pineapple into cubes.

   - Halve the strawberries.

2. Thread the fruit onto the skewers, alternating the different types of fruit.

Storage Instructions:
- Serve the fruit kabobs immediately for best quality and texture.
- If you have any lefover fruit, store it in an airtight container in the refrigerator for up to 3 days.

Tips:
- Encourage the 9-year-old to help assemble the fruit kabobs for a fun, interactive activity.

- Provide a variety of colorful fruits to make the kabobs visually appealing.

- Consider offering a yogurt-based dipping sauce on the side for extra flavor.

- Adjust the fruit selection based on the 9-year-old's preferences.

Nutrition Information:
Calories: 80 | Total Fat: 0g | Saturated Fat: 0g | Cholesterol: 0mg | Sodium: 0mg | Total Carbohydrates: 20g | Dietary Fiber: 2g | Total Sugars: 16g | Protein: 1g

Snacks (23 Recipes)

29. Mini Rice Cakes with Almond Butter

Ingredients:
- 2 mini rice cakes
- 2 tablespoons creamy almond butter
- 1 tablespoon sliced strawberries (optional)

Equipment:
- Plate
- Knife

Directions:
1. Spread the almond butter evenly over the rice cakes.

2. If desired, top the almond butter with sliced strawberries.

Storage Instructions:
- This snack is best served immediately, but any leftover rice cakes can be stored in an airtight container at room temperature for up to 3 days.

Tips:
- Encourage the 9-year-old to help assemble the snack for a fun, interactive experience.

- Offer a variety of toppings, such as banana slices, honey, or cinnamon, to keep the snack interesting.

- Adjust the amount of almond butter based on the 9-year-old's preferences.

- Provide a small glass of milk or water to accompany the snack.

Nutrition Information:
Calories: 150 | Total Fat: 9g | Saturated Fat: 1g | Cholesterol: 0mg | Sodium: 100mg | Total Carbohydrates: 14g | Dietary Fiber: 2g | Total Sugars: 3g | Protein: 5g

PreparationTime: 5 minutes
Cook Time: 0 minutes
Total Time: 5 minutes
Serves: 1

30. Popcorn with Parmesan

Ingredients:
- 1/4 cup popcorn kernels
- 2 tablespoons olive oil
- 1/4 cup grated Parmesan cheese
- 1/2 teaspoon garlic powder
- 1/4 teaspoon salt

PreparationTime: 5 minutes
Cook Time: 5 minutes
Total Time: 10 minutes
Serves: 4

Equipment:
- Large pot with lid
- Microwave-safe bowl (optional)
- Measuring cups and spoons

Directions:

1. In a large pot with a lid, heat the olive oil over medium-high heat.

2. Add the popcorn kernels and cover the pot. Cook, shaking the pot occasionally, until the popping slows to 2-3 seconds between pops.

3. Remove the pot from the heat and transfer the popped popcorn to a large bowl.

4. Sprinkle the Parmesan cheese, garlic powder, and salt over the popcorn and toss to coat evenly.

Storage Instructions:
- Store the popcorn in an airtight container at room temperature for up to 3 days.

Tips:
- For a microwave version, place the popcorn kernels in a microwave-safe bowl and cook on high for 2-3 minutes, or until the popping slows.

- Experiment with different seasonings, such as chili powder, paprika, or dried herbs.

- Adjust the amount of Parmesan cheese to your taste preference.

Nutrition Information:
Calories: 150 | Total Fat: 10g | Saturated Fat: 2g | Cholesterol: 5mg | Sodium: 300mg | Total Carbohydrates: 12g | Dietary Fiber: 2g | Total Sugars: 0g | Protein: 5g

Snacks (23 Recipes)

31. Frozen Yogurt Bites

Ingredients:
- 1 cup plain Greek yogurt
- 2 tablespoons honey
- 1/2 cup fresh or frozen berries
(such as blueberries, raspberries, or strawberries)

PreparationTime: 10 minutes
Freeze Time: 2-3 hours
Total Time: 2-3 hours 10 minutes
Serves: 12 bites

Equipment:
- Mini muffin tin or silicone mold
- Spoon
- Parchment paper or silicone baking mat

Directions:
1. In a small bowl, mix the Greek yogurt and honey until well combined.

2. Line a mini muffin tin or silicone mold with parchment paper or a silicone baking mat.

3. Spoon the yogurt mixture evenly into the muffin cups or mold, filling them about 3/4 full.

4. Gently press 1-2 berries into the center of each yogurt bite.

5. Place the muffin tin or mold in the freezer and freeze for 2-3 hours, or until the yogurt bites are completely frozen.

6. Once frozen, remove the yogurt bites from the mold and store them in an airtight container in the freezer.

Storage Instructions:
- Store the frozen yogurt bites in an airtight container in the freezer for up to 2 months.

Tips:
- Encourage the 9-year-old to help with the mixing and assembly of the yogurt bites.
- Experiment with different fruit combinations, such as diced mango, kiwi, or pineapple.
- For a creamier texture, use full-fat Greek yogurt instead of low-fat.
- Serve the frozen yogurt bites as a healthy, refreshing snack on a hot day.

Nutrition Information:
Calories: 40 | Total Fat: 1g | Saturated Fat: 0g | Cholesterol: 5mg | Sodium: 15mg | Total Carbohydrates: 6g | Dietary Fiber: 1g | Total Sugars: 5g | Protein: 3g

Snacks (23 Recipes)

32. Granola Bars

Ingredients:
- 2 cups old-fashioned oats
- 1/2 cup sliced almonds
- 1/2 cup shredded coconut
- 1/4 cup honey
- 1/4 cup brown sugar
- 1/4 cup peanut butter
- 1 teaspoon vanilla extract
- 1/4 teaspoon salt

PreparationTime: 15 minutes
Cook Time: 25 minutes
Total Time: 40 minutes
Serves: 12 bars

Equipment:
- 8x8-inch baking pan
- Mixing bowl
- Spatula
- Parchment paper

Directions:
1. Preheat the oven to 325°F (165°C). Line an 8x8-inch baking pan with parchment paper, leaving some overhang on the sides for easy removal.
2. In a large mixing bowl, combine the oats, almonds, and shredded coconut.
3. In a small saucepan, heat the honey, brown sugar, and peanut butter over medium heat, stirring constantly, until the mixture is smooth and well combined.
4. Remove the honey mixture from the heat and stir in the vanilla extract and salt.
5. Pour the honey mixture over the oat mixture and stir until the oats are evenly coated.
6. Transfer the mixture to the prepared baking pan and press it down firmly to create an even layer.
7. Bake for 25 minutes, or until the edges are lightly golden.
8. Allow the granola bars to cool completely in the pan before lifting them out using the parchment paper overhang.
9. Cut the granola bars into 12 equal pieces.

Storage Instructions:
- Store the granola bars in an airtight container at room temperature for up to 1 week.

Tips:
- Encourage the 9-year-old to help measure and mix the ingredients.
- Experiment with different mix-ins, such as dried fruit, chocolate chips, or seeds, to customize the granola bars.
- Cut the granola bars into fun shapes or smaller pieces for easy snacking.
- Serve the granola bars with a glass of milk or a piece of fresh fruit for a balanced snack.

Nutrition Information:
Calories: 170 | Total Fat: 8g | Saturated Fat: 2g | Cholesterol: 0mg | Sodium: 75mg | Total Carbohydrates: 22g | Dietary Fiber: 3g | Total Sugars: 10g | Protein: 4g

Snacks (23 Recipes)

33. Veggie Chips

Ingredients:
- 2 medium zucchini, sliced into 1/8-inch thick rounds
- 2 medium carrots, sliced into 1/8-inch thick rounds
- 1 medium sweet potato, sliced into 1/8-inch thick rounds
- 2 tablespoons olive oil
- 1/2 teaspoon salt
- 1/4 teaspoon black pepper

PreparationTime: 15 minutes
Cook Time: 20-25 minutes
Total Time: 35-40 minutes
Serves: 4

Equipment:
- 2 baking sheets
- Parchment paper or silicone baking mats
- Mandoline slicer or sharp knife (for slicing the vegetables)

Directions:
1. Preheat the oven to 375°F (190°C).
2. Line two baking sheets with parchment paper or silicone baking mats.
3. Slice the zucchini, carrots, and sweet potato into 1/8-inch thick rounds using a mandoline slicer or a sharp knife.
4. In a large bowl, toss the vegetable slices with the olive oil, salt, and black pepper until evenly coated.
5. Arrange the vegetable slices in a single layer on the prepared baking sheets, making sure they are not overlapping.
6. Bake for 20-25 minutes, flipping the slices halfway through, until they are crispy and lightly browned.
7. Remove the baking sheets from the oven and let the veggie chips cool completely before serving.

Storage Instructions:
- Store the cooled veggie chips in an airtight container at room temperature for up to 5 days.

Tips:
- Encourage the 9-year-old to help with the vegetable slicing and tossing.
- Experiment with different vegetable combinations, such as beets, parsnips, or radishes.
- Sprinkle the veggie chips with additional seasonings, such as garlic powder, paprika, or Parmesan cheese, for extra flavor.
- Serve the veggie chips as a healthy alternative to traditional potato chips.

Nutrition Information:
Calories: 80 | Total Fat: 4g | Saturated Fat: 0.5g | Cholesterol: 0mg | Sodium: 230mg | Total Carbohydrates: 10g | Dietary Fiber: 2g | Total Sugars: 3g | Protein: 1g

Snacks (23 Recipes)

34. Banana Bread Slices

Ingredients:
- 1 3/4 cups all-purpose flour
- 1 teaspoon baking soda
- 1/4 teaspoon salt
- 1/2 cup unsalted butter, softened
- 3/4 cup granulated sugar
- 2 large eggs
- 1 teaspoon vanilla extract
- 3 ripe bananas, mashed (about 1 cup)

Equipment:
- Loaf pan
- Mixing bowls
- Electric mixer or whisk
- Measuring cups and spoons
- Knife and cutting board

PreparationTime: 15 minutes
Cook Time: 55 minutes
Total Time: 1 hour 10 minutes
Serves: 12 slices

Directions:
1. Preheat the oven to 350°F (175°C). Grease a 9x5-inch loaf pan.
2. In a medium bowl, whisk together the flour, baking soda, and salt.
3. In a large bowl, beat the butter and sugar with an electric mixer until light and fluffy, about 2-3 minutes.
4. Add the eggs one at a time, beating well after each addition. Stir in the vanilla and mashed bananas.
5. Gradually add the dry ingredients to the wet ingredients, mixing just until combined.
6. Pour the batter into the prepared loaf pan and bake for 55-60 minutes, or until a toothpick inserted into the center comes out clean.
7. Allow the banana bread to cool in the pan for 10 minutes, then transfer to a wire rack to cool completely. Slice the banana bread and serve.

Storage Instructions:
- Store the banana bread slices in an airtight container at room temperature for up to 4 days, or in the refrigerator for up to 1 week.

Tips:
- Encourage the 9-year-old to help mash the bananas and mix the batter.
- Serve the banana bread slices with a glass of milk or a small scoop of vanilla ice cream for a special treat.
- Experiment with add-ins like chocolate chips, chopped nuts, or cinnamon to customize the flavor.

Nutrition Information:
Calories: 200 | Total Fat: 8g | Saturated Fat: 5g | Cholesterol: 45mg | Sodium: 170mg | Total Carbohydrates: 30g | Dietary Fiber: 2g | Total Sugars: 15g | Protein: 3g

Snacks (23 Recipes)

35. Celery Sticks with Cream Cheese

Ingredients:
- 2-3 celery stalks, cut into 3-inch sticks
- 2 tablespoons cream cheese, softened

Equipment:
- Cutting board
- Knife
- Plate

Directions:
1. Wash the celery stalks and cut them into 3-inch sticks.

2. Spread the cream cheese evenly onto the celery sticks.

Storage Instructions:
- This snack is best served immediately, but any leftover celery sticks can be stored in an airtight container in the refrigerator for up to 3 days.

Tips:
- Encourage the 9-year-old to help with the celery preparation and assembly of the snack.

- Offer a variety of cream cheese flavors, such as plain, garlic, or herb, to keep it interesting.

- Provide a small container of raisins or dried cranberries to add as a topping, if desired.

- Serve the celery sticks with a glass of milk or water for a balanced snack.

Nutrition Information:
Calories: 60 | Total Fat: 4g | Saturated Fat: 2.5g | Cholesterol: 15mg | Sodium: 120mg | Total Carbohydrates: 4g | Dietary Fiber: 1g | Total Sugars: 2g | Protein: 2g

PreparationTime: 10 minutes
Cook Time: 0 minutes
Total Time: 10 minutes
Serves: 1

Snacks (23 Recipes)

36. Edamame

Ingredients:
- 1/2 cup frozen edamame, in the pod
- 1/4 teaspoon sea salt (optional)

Equipment:
- Pot with steamer basket or saucepan
- Bowl

PreparationTime: 5 minutes
Cook Time: 5 minutes
Total Time: 10 minutes
Serves: 1

Directions:
1. Bring a pot of water to a boil. Place the frozen edamame in a steamer basket and steam for 5 minutes, or until the pods are bright green and tender.

2. Alternatively, you can boil the edamame in the pot of water for 5 minutes.

3. Drain the edamame and transfer to a bowl. Sprinkle with sea salt, if desired.

Storage Instructions:
- Cooked edamame can be stored in an airtight container in the refrigerator for up to 3 days.

Tips:
- Encourage the 9-year-old to help with the preparation and seasoning of the edamame.

- Provide a small bowl of soy sauce or lemon wedges for dipping, if desired.

- Edamame can be served warm or at room temperature.

- Discuss the nutritional benefits of edamame, such as its high protein and fiber content.

Nutrition Information:
Calories: 100 | Total Fat: 5g | Saturated Fat: 0.5g | Cholesterol: 0mg | Sodium: 95mg | Total Carbohydrates: 8g | Dietary Fiber: 4g | Total Sugars: 2g | Protein: 10g

37. Hard-Boiled Eggs

Ingredients:
- 4 large eggs

Equipment:
- Saucepan with lid
- Spoon
- Bowl of ice water

PreparationTime: 10 minutes
Cook Time: 12 minutes
Total Time: 22 minutes
Serves: 4 eggs

Directions:

1. Place the eggs in a single layer in a saucepan and cover with cold water by 1 inch.

2. Bring the water to a boil over high heat.

3. Once the water is boiling, remove the pan from the heat, cover, and let the eggs sit for 12 minutes.

4. Carefully drain the hot water and cover the eggs with cold water. Let them sit in the ice water for 5 minutes.

5. Gently tap the eggs on the counter to crack the shells, then peel them under running water.

Storage Instructions:
- Store the peeled hard-boiled eggs in an airtight container in the refrigerator for up to 1 week.

Tips:
- Encourage the 9-year-old to help with the peeling process.
- Provide a small bowl of salt, pepper, or other seasonings for the 9-year-old to customize the eggs.
- Serve the hard-boiled eggs as a protein-rich snack, or use them in other recipes, such as egg salad or deviled eggs.
- Discuss the nutritional benefits of eggs, including their high-quality protein and essential vitamins and minerals.

Nutrition Information:
Calories: 70 | Total Fat: 5g | Saturated Fat: 2g | Cholesterol: 185mg | Sodium: 70mg | Total Carbohydrates: 0g | Dietary Fiber: 0g | Total Sugars: 0g | Protein: 6g

Snacks (23 Recipes)

38. Homemade Fruit Leather

Ingredients:
- 2 cups pureed fruit (such as strawberries, mango, or mixed berries)
- 1-2 tablespoons honey or maple syrup (optional)

PreparationTime: 15 minutes
Cook Time: 6-8 hours
Total Time: 6-8 hours 15 minutes
Serves: 8-10 pieces

Equipment:
- Blender or food processor
- Parchment paper or silicone baking mat
- Baking sheet
- Scissors or knife (for cutting the fruit leather)

Directions:

1. Preheat your oven to the lowest setting, usually around 135°F (57°C).

2. In a blender or food processor, puree the fruit until smooth.

3. If desired, stir in 1-2 tablespoons of honey or maple syrup to sweeten the fruit puree.

4. Line a baking sheet with parchment paper or a silicone baking mat.

5. Spread the fruit puree evenly over the prepared baking sheet, making sure it's about 1/4 inch thick.

6. Place the baking sheet in the preheated oven and let the fruit leather dry for 6-8 hours, or until it's no longer tacky to the touch.

7. Remove the baking sheet from the oven and let the fruit leather cool completely.

8. Peel the fruit leather off the parchment paper or silicone mat.

9. Using scissors or a knife, cut the fruit leather into strips or shapes.

Storage Instructions:
- Store the homemade fruit leather in an airtight container at room temperature for up to 2 weeks.

Tips:
- Encourage the 9-year-old to help with the fruit selection and puree preparation.
- Experiment with different fruit combinations to find their favorite flavors.
- Cut the fruit leather into fun shapes or small pieces for easy snacking.
- Provide the fruit leather as a healthy alternative to store-bought fruit snacks.

Nutrition Information:
Calories: 50 | Total Fat: 0g | Saturated Fat: 0g | Cholesterol: 0mg | Sodium: 0mg | Total Carbohydrates: 13g | Dietary Fiber: 1g | Total Sugars: 11g | Protein: 0g

Snacks (23 Recipes)

39. Smoothie Popsicles

Ingredients:
- 1 cup frozen mixed berries (such as strawberries, blueberries, and raspberries)
- 1 cup plain Greek yogurt
- 1/2 cup milk (dairy, almond, or oat)
- 2 tablespoons honey (optional)

PreparationTime: 10 minutes
Freeze Time: 4-6 hours
Total Time: 4-6 hours 10 minutes
Serves: 6 popsicles

Equipment:
- Blender
- Popsicle molds or small paper cups with popsicle sticks

Directions:

1. In a blender, combine the frozen mixed berries, Greek yogurt, milk, and honey (if using).

2. Blend the ingredients until smooth and creamy.

3. Carefully pour the smoothie mixture into popsicle molds or small paper cups.

4. Insert popsicle sticks into the center of each mold or cup.

5. Place the popsicle molds or cups in the freezer and freeze for 4-6 hours, or until completely frozen.

6. Once frozen, remove the popsicles from the molds or cups and serve.

Storage Instructions:
- Store the frozen smoothie popsicles in an airtight container in the freezer for up to 2 months.

Tips:
- Encourage the 9-year-old to help with the blending and pouring of the smoothie mixture.
- Experiment with different fruit combinations, such as mango and pineapple or banana and spinach, to create a variety of flavors.
- For a creamier texture, use full-fat Greek yogurt instead of low-fat.
- Serve the smoothie popsicles as a refreshing and healthy treat on a hot day.

Nutrition Information:
Calories: 90 | Total Fat: 2g | Saturated Fat: 1g | Cholesterol: 5mg | Sodium: 35mg | Total Carbohydrates: 14g | Dietary Fiber: 2g | Total Sugars: 11g | Protein: 5g

40. Mini Pita Pizzas

Ingredients:
- 4 mini whole wheat pita breads
- 1/2 cup tomato sauce
- 1 cup shredded mozzarella cheese
- 1/4 cup sliced pepperoni (optional)
- 1/4 cup chopped bell peppers (optional)
- 1/4 cup sliced mushrooms (optional)

PreparationTime: 10 minutes
Cook Time: 10 minutes
Total Time: 20 minutes
Serves: 4 mini pizzas

Equipment:
- Baking sheet
- Knife
- Spoon

Directions:
1. Preheat the oven to 400°F (200°C).

2. Place the mini pita breads on a baking sheet.

3. Spread the tomato sauce evenly over the pita breads.

4. Sprinkle the shredded mozzarella cheese over the sauce.

5. If desired, top the pizzas with pepperoni, bell peppers, and/or mushrooms.

6. Bake the mini pita pizzas for 10 minutes, or until the cheese is melted and bubbly.

7. Remove the pizzas from the oven and let them cool for a few minutes before serving.

Storage Instructions:
- Any leftover mini pita pizzas can be stored in an airtight container in the refrigerator for up to 3 days.

Tips:
- Encourage the 9-year-old to help with the assembly of the mini pizzas, such as adding the toppings.
- Offer a variety of vegetable toppings to encourage healthy eating.
- Serve the mini pita pizzas with a side salad or fresh fruit for a balanced meal.
- Discuss the importance of portion control and moderation when it comes to pizza and other treats.

Nutrition Information:
Calories: 200 | Total Fat: 8g | Saturated Fat: 4g | Cholesterol: 20mg | Sodium: 450mg | Total Carbohydrates: 20g | Dietary Fiber: 3g | Total Sugars: 4g | Protein: 12g

Snacks (23 Recipes)

41. Cheese Quesadillas

Ingredients:
- 4 small whole wheat tortillas
- 1 cup shredded cheddar or Monterey Jack cheese
- 2 tablespoons salsa (optional)
- 2 tablespoons sour cream (optional)

Equipment:
- Skillet or griddle
- Spatula
- Cutting board
- Knife

PreparationTime: 10 minutes
Cook Time: 10 minutes
Total Time: 20 minutes
Serves: 2 quesadillas

Directions:

1. Heat a skillet or griddle over medium heat.

2. Place one tortilla in the skillet and sprinkle half of the shredded cheese over one side of the tortilla.

3. Fold the tortilla in half to create a half-moon shape.

4. Cook the quesadilla for 2-3 minutes per side, or until the cheese is melted and the tortilla is lightly browned.

5. Repeat steps 2-4 with the remaining tortilla and cheese to make the second quesadilla.

6. Cut each quesadilla into halves or quarters.

7. Serve the cheese quesadillas with salsa and sour cream, if desired.

Storage Instructions:
- Any leftover quesadillas can be stored in an airtight container in the refrigerator for up to 3 days.

Tips:
- Encourage the 9-year-old to help with the assembly and cooking of the quesadillas.
- Offer a variety of fillings, such as diced chicken, black beans, or sautéed vegetables, to customize the quesadillas.
- Serve the quesadillas with a side of fresh fruit or a small salad for a balanced meal.
- Discuss the importance of portion control and moderation when it comes to cheese and other dairy products.

Nutrition Information:
Calories: 300 | Total Fat: 15g | Saturated Fat: 8g | Cholesterol: 40mg | Sodium: 550mg | Total Carbohydrates: 28g | Dietary Fiber: 4g | Total Sugars: 2g | Protein: 15g

Snacks (23 Recipes)

42. Greek Yogurt with Honey

Ingredients:
- 1 cup plain Greek yogurt
- 1-2 tablespoons honey
- 1/4 cup fresh berries (such as blueberries, raspberries, or strawberries)

Equipment:
- Bowl
- Spoon

Directions:
1. Place the Greek yogurt in a bowl.

2. Drizzle the honey over the yogurt, using 1-2 tablespoons depending on the 9-year-old's preference.

3. Top the yogurt and honey with the fresh berries.

Storage Instructions:
- This snack is best served immediately, but any leftover yogurt can be stored in an airtight container in the refrigerator for up to 3 days.

Tips:
- Encourage the 9-year-old to help measure and assemble the ingredients.
- Offer a variety of fresh fruit options to allow the 9-year-old to customize the snack.
- Discuss the nutritional benefits of Greek yogurt, such as its high protein and calcium content.
- Serve the yogurt with a small spoon or provide a spoon for the 9-year-old to use.

Nutrition Information:
Calories: 180 | Total Fat: 5g | Saturated Fat: 3g | Cholesterol: 20mg | Sodium: 65mg | Total Carbohydrates: 22g | Dietary Fiber: 2g | Total Sugars: 18g | Protein: 15g

PreparationTime: 5 minutes
Cook Time: 0 minutes
Total Time: 5 minutes
Serves: 1

Snacks (23 Recipes)

43. Mini Sandwich Roll-Ups

Ingredients:
- 4 slices whole wheat bread
- 2 tablespoons cream cheese, softened
- 2 tablespoons shredded cheddar cheese
- 2 tablespoons diced cucumber
- 2 tablespoons diced bell pepper

PreparationTime: 10 minutes
Cook Time: 0 minutes
Total Time: 10 minutes
Serves: 4 roll-ups

Equipment:
- Cutting board
- Knife
- Toothpicks or skewers (optional)

Directions:

1. Using a rolling pin, gently roll the bread slices to flatten them and make them more pliable.

2. Spread the cream cheese evenly over the surface of each bread slice.

3. Sprinkle the shredded cheddar cheese, diced cucumber, and diced bell pepper over the cream cheese.

4. Carefully roll up each bread slice tightly, starting from one of the shorter sides..

5. Secure the roll-ups with toothpicks or skewers, if desired.

6. Cut each roll-up into 2-3 pieces.

Storage Instructions:
- Store the mini sandwich roll-ups in an airtight container in the refrigerator for up to 3 days.

Tips:
- Encourage the 9-year-old to help with the assembly of the roll-ups, such as spreading the cream cheese and adding the fillings.
- Experiment with different fillings, such as sliced turkey, hummus, or shredded carrots, to keep the roll-ups interesting.
- Cut the roll-ups into smaller pieces for easier handling and snacking.
- Serve the mini sandwich roll-ups as a fun and portable lunch or snack option.

Nutrition Information:
Calories: 100 | Total Fat: 5g | Saturated Fat: 3g | Cholesterol: 15mg | Sodium: 200mg | Total Carbohydrates: 10g | Dietary Fiber: 2g | Total Sugars: 2g | Protein: 5g

Snacks (23 Recipes)

44. Zucchini Muffins

Ingredients:
- 1 1/2 cups all-purpose flour
- 1 teaspoon baking soda
- 1/2 teaspoon ground cinnamon
- 1/4 teaspoon salt
- 1 cup grated zucchini (about 1 medium zucchini)
- 1/2 cup granulated sugar
- 1/4 cup vegetable oil
- 1 large egg
- 1 teaspoon vanilla extract

PreparationTime: 15 minutes
Cook Time: 20-25 minutes
Total Time: 35-40 minutes
Serves: 12 muffins

Equipment:
- Muffin tin
- Mixing bowls
- Grater
- Spoon
- Whisk

Directions:
1. Preheat the oven to 350°F (175°C). Grease a 12-cup muffin tin or line it with paper liners.
2. In a medium bowl, whisk together the flour, baking soda, cinnamon, and salt.
3. In a separate bowl, combine the grated zucchini, sugar, vegetable oil, egg, and vanilla extract. Mix well.
4. Gently fold the wet ingredients into the dry ingredients until just combined, being careful not to overmix.
5. Divide the batter evenly among the prepared muffin cups, filling them about 3/4 full.
6. Bake for 20-25 minutes, or until a toothpick inserted into the center comes out clean.
7. Allow the muffins to cool in the tin for 5 minutes, then transfer them to a wire rack to cool completely.

Storage Instructions:
- Store the zucchini muffins in an airtight container at room temperature for up to 3 days, or in the refrigerator for up to 1 week.

Tips:
- Encourage the 9-year-old to help with the grating of the zucchini and the mixing of the batter.
- Experiment with different mix-ins, such as chopped walnuts, chocolate chips, or dried cranberries, to customize the muffins.
- Serve the zucchini muffins as a healthy snack or breakfast option.
- Discuss the nutritional benefits of zucchini, such as its high fiber and vitamin content.

Nutrition Information:
Calories: 150 | Total Fat: 6g | Saturated Fat: 1g | Cholesterol: 20mg | Sodium: 180mg | Total Carbohydrates: 22g | Dietary Fiber: 1g | Total Sugars: 10g | Protein: 2g

Snacks (23 Recipes)

45. Baked Sweet Potato Fries

Ingredients:
- 2 medium sweet potatoes, peeled and cut into 1/2-inch thick fries
- 2 tablespoons olive oil
- 1/2 teaspoon garlic powder
- 1/2 teaspoon paprika
- 1/4 teaspoon salt

PreparationTime: 15 minutes
Cook Time: 25-30 minutes
Total Time: 40-45 minutes
Serves: 4

Equipment:
- Baking sheet
- Parchment paper or silicone baking mat
- Cutting board
- Knife

Directions:

1. Preheat the oven to 400°F (200°C).

2. Line a baking sheet with parchment paper or a silicone baking mat.

3. Peel the sweet potatoes and cut them into 1/2-inch thick fries.

4. In a large bowl, toss the sweet potato fries with the olive oil, garlic powder, paprika, and salt until evenly coated.

5. Spread the fries in a single layer on the prepared baking sheet, making sure they are not touching each other.

6. Bake for 25-30 minutes, flipping the fries halfway through, until they are crispy and golden brown.

7. Remove the baked sweet potato fries from the oven and let them cool for a few minutes before serving.

Storage Instructions:
- Store any leftover baked sweet potato fries in an airtight container in the refrigerator for up to 3 days.

Tips:
- Encourage the 9-year-old to help with the peeling and cutting of the sweet potatoes.
- Experiment with different seasoning blends, such as chili powder, cumin, or Italian herbs.
- Serve the baked sweet potato fries with a side of ketchup, ranch dressing, or honey mustard for dipping.
- Discuss the nutritional benefits of sweet potatoes, including their high vitamin A and fiber content.

Nutrition Information:
Calories: 120 | Total Fat: 5g | Saturated Fat: 1g | Cholesterol: 0mg | Sodium: 180mg | Total Carbohydrates: 17g | Dietary Fiber: 3g | Total Sugars: 5g | Protein: 2g

Snacks (23 Recipes)

46. Pretzel Sticks with Cheese Dip

Ingredients:
- 8-10 whole grain pretzel sticks
- 2 tablespoons shredded cheddar cheese
- 1 tablespoon milk
- 1/2 teaspoon cornstarch

PreparationTime: 10 minutes
Cook Time: 0 minutes
Total Time: 10 minutes
Serves: 1

Equipment:
- Small saucepan
- Spoon
- Plate

Directions:
1. In a small saucepan, combine the shredded cheddar cheese, milk, and cornstarch.

2. Heat the mixture over medium-low heat, stirring constantly, until the cheese is melted and the dip is smooth and creamy, about 2-3 minutes.

3. Remove the cheese dip from the heat and transfer it to a small bowl or ramekin.

4. Arrange the pretzel sticks on a plate and serve them alongside the warm cheese dip.

Storage Instructions:
- Any leftover cheese dip can be stored in an airtight container in the refrigerator for up to 3 days.

Tips:
- Encourage the 9-year-old to help with the assembly and dipping of the pretzel sticks.
- Offer a variety of dipping options, such as hummus or ranch dressing, to provide different flavors.
- Discuss the importance of portion control and moderation when it comes to snacks and dips.
- Serve the pretzel sticks and cheese dip as a fun and interactive snack.

Nutrition Information:
Calories: 150 | Total Fat: 7g | Saturated Fat: 4g | Cholesterol: 20mg | Sodium: 450mg | Total Carbohydrates: 16g | Dietary Fiber: 2g | Total Sugars: 1g | Protein: 7g

47. Turkey and Cheese Sandwich

Ingredients:
- 2 slices whole wheat bread
- 2 slices turkey breast
- 1 slice cheddar or Swiss cheese
- 1 teaspoon mustard (optional)
- 1 teaspoon mayonnaise (optional)

PreparationTime: 5 minutes
Cook Time: 0 minutes
Total Time: 5 minutes
Serves: 1 sandwich

Equipment:
- Cutting board
- Knife

Directions:

1. Lay the two slices of whole wheat bread on a clean surface.

2. Spread the mustard (if using) on one slice of bread and the mayonnaise (if using) on the other slice.

3. Place the two slices of turkey on one slice of bread.

4. Top the turkey with the slice of cheese.

5. Place the other slice of bread on top to create a sandwich.

Storage Instructions:
- Wrap the sandwich tightly in plastic wrap or foil and store in the refrigerator for up to 3 days.

Tips:
- Encourage the 9-year-old to help with the assembly of the sandwich.
- Offer a variety of condiments, such as honey mustard or avocado spread, to customize the sandwich.
- Serve the sandwich with a side of fresh fruit, carrot sticks, or a small salad for a balanced meal.
- Discuss the importance of choosing whole grain breads and lean proteins for a healthy diet.

Nutrition Information:
Calories: 300 | Total Fat: 10g | Saturated Fat: 4g | Cholesterol: 45mg | Sodium: 650mg | Total Carbohydrates: 30g | Dietary Fiber: 4g | Total Sugars: 4g | Protein: 22g

48. Chicken Salad Wrap

Ingredients:
- 1/2 cup cooked, shredded chicken
- 2 tablespoons plain Greek yogurt
- 1 tablespoon diced celery
- 1 tablespoon diced red onion
- 1 teaspoon Dijon mustard
- 1/4 teaspoon dried dill (optional)
- Salt and pepper to taste
- 1 whole wheat tortilla or wrap

PreparationTime: 15 minutes
Cook Time: 0 minutes
Total Time: 15 minutes
Serves: 1 wrap

Equipment:
- Mixing bowl
- Spoon
- Knife
- Cutting board

Directions:

1. In a mixing bowl, combine the shredded chicken, Greek yogurt, diced celery, diced red onion, Dijon mustard, and dried dill (if using). Mix well.

2. Season the chicken salad with salt and pepper to taste.

3. Lay the whole wheat tortilla or wrap on a flat surface.

4. Spoon the chicken salad mixture onto the center of the tortilla.

5. Fold the bottom of the tortilla up over the filling, then fold in the sides and continue rolling up tightly to create a wrap.

Storage Instructions:
- Wrap the chicken salad wrap tightly in plastic wrap or foil and store in the refrigerator for up to 3 days.

Tips:
- Encourage the 9-year-old to help with the mixing and assembly of the wrap.
- Offer a variety of crunchy vegetables, such as shredded carrots or sliced cucumber, to add to the chicken salad.
- Provide a small side of fresh fruit or a handful of whole grain crackers to accompany the wrap.
- Discuss the importance of protein and healthy fats in a balanced diet.

Nutrition Information:
Calories: 250 | Total Fat: 8g | Saturated Fat: 2g | Cholesterol: 55mg | Sodium: 450mg | Total Carbohydrates: 22g | Dietary Fiber: 3g | Total Sugars: 3g | Protein: 22g

Lunches (23 Recipes)

49. Veggie Pasta Salad

Ingredients:
- 2 cups cooked whole wheat pasta, cooled
- 1/2 cup diced cucumber
- 1/2 cup diced cherry tomatoes
- 1/4 cup diced bell pepper
- 2 tablespoons diced red onion
- 2 tablespoons Italian dressing
- 1 tablespoon grated Parmesan cheese (optional)
- Salt and pepper to taste

PreparationTime: 20 minutes
Cook Time: 10 minutes
Total Time: 30 minutes
Serves: 4

Equipment:
- Pot for cooking pasta
- Cutting board
- Knife
- Large mixing bowl
- Spoon

Directions:
1. Cook the whole wheat pasta according to the package instructions. Drain and rinse with cold water to cool completely.
2. In a large mixing bowl, combine the cooked and cooled pasta, diced cucumber, cherry tomatoes, bell pepper, and red onion.
3. Drizzle the Italian dressing over the pasta and vegetables, and gently toss to coat everything evenly.
4. If desired, sprinkle the grated Parmesan cheese over the salad.
5. Season with salt and pepper to taste.

Storage Instructions:
- Store the veggie pasta salad in an airtight container in the refrigerator for up to 3 days.

Tips:
- Encourage the 9-year-old to help with the chopping of the vegetables and the assembly of the salad.
- Experiment with different vegetables, such as shredded carrots, diced zucchini, or halved snap peas, to keep the salad interesting.
- Offer the pasta salad as a side dish or a light main course, accompanied by a piece of grilled chicken or a hard-boiled egg for added protein.
- Discuss the importance of incorporating a variety of colorful fruits and vegetables into a balanced diet.

Nutrition Information:
Calories: 150 | Total Fat: 5g | Saturated Fat: 1g | Cholesterol: 0mg | Sodium: 200mg | Total Carbohydrates: 22g | Dietary Fiber: 3g | Total Sugars: 3g | Protein: 6g

Lunches (23 Recipes)

50. Mini Meatball Subs

Ingredients:
- 12 frozen pre-cooked meatballs
- 1/2 cup marinara sauce
- 4 small whole wheat rolls or slider buns, split in half
- 1/2 cup shredded mozzarella cheese

PreparationTime: 20 minutes
Cook Time: 15 minutes
Total Time: 35 minutes
Serves: 4 mini subs

Equipment:
- Baking sheet
- Skillet or saucepan
- Spoon

Directions:

1. Preheat the oven to 375°F (190°C).

2. In a skillet or saucepan, heat the marinara sauce over medium heat.

3. Add the frozen meatballs to the sauce and simmer for 10-15 minutes, or until the meatballs are heated through.

4. Place the split rolls or buns on a baking sheet.

5. Top each bottom half of the rolls with 3 meatballs and a spoonful of the marinara sauce.

6. Sprinkle the shredded mozzarella cheese over the meatballs.

7. Bake the mini meatball subs for 5-7 minutes, or until the cheese is melted and bubbly.

8. Remove the subs from the oven and place the top halves of the rolls on the meatballs.

Storage Instructions:
- Any leftover mini meatball subs can be stored in an airtight container in the refrigerator for up to 3 days.

Tips:
- Encourage the 9-year-old to help with the assembly of the mini subs, such as placing the meatballs and sprinkling the cheese.
- Offer a side of fresh vegetables, such as carrot sticks or celery, to balance the meal.
- Discuss the importance of portion control and moderation when it comes to processed meats and high-sodium foods.
- Provide a small bowl of grated Parmesan cheese or dried oregano for the 9-year-old to customize the subs.

Nutrition Information:
Calories: 250 | Total Fat: 10g | Saturated Fat: 4g | Cholesterol: 45mg | Sodium: 650mg | Total Carbohydrates: 25g | Dietary Fiber: 3g | Total Sugars: 5g | Protein: 15g

Lunches (23 Recipes)

51. Quinoa Salad with Veggies

Ingredients:
- 1 cup quinoa, rinsed
- 2 cups vegetable broth
- 1 cup diced cucumber
- 1 cup diced tomatoes
- 1/2 cup diced red onion
- 1/2 cup diced bell pepper
- 1/4 cup chopped fresh parsley
- 2 tablespoons olive oil
- 2 tablespoons lemon juice
- 1 teaspoon Dijon mustard
- Salt and pepper to taste

Equipment:
- Saucepan
- Cutting board - Knife
- Large bowl - Whisk

PreparationTime: 15 minutes
Cook Time: 20 minutes
Total Time: 35 minutes
Serves: 4

Directions:
1. In a saucepan, combine the quinoa and vegetable broth. Bring to a boil, then reduce heat to low, cover, and simmer for 15-20 minutes, or until the quinoa is tender and the liquid is absorbed.
2. Transfer the cooked quinoa to a large bowl and let it cool slightly.
3. Add the diced cucumber, tomatoes, red onion, bell pepper, and chopped parsley to the bowl with the quinoa.
4. In a small bowl, whisk together the olive oil, lemon juice, and Dijon mustard. Season with salt and pepper.
5. Pour the dressing over the quinoa and vegetable mixture and toss gently to combine.
6. Serve chilled or at room temperature.

Storage Instructions: - Store the quinoa salad in an airtight container in the refrigerator for up to 4 days.

Tips:
- Feel free to add other vegetables or herbs to the salad, such as diced avocado, feta cheese, or fresh basil.
- For a heartier meal, you can add grilled chicken or shrimp to the salad.
- Quinoa can be cooked in advance and stored in the refrigerator for up to 5 days, making this salad a quick and easy option.

Nutrition Information: Calories: 220 | Total Fat: 9g | Saturated Fat: 1g | Cholesterol: 0mg | Sodium: 320mg | Total Carbohydrates: 30g | Dietary Fiber: 4g | Total Sugars: 3g | Protein: 6g

Lunches (23 Recipes)

52. Grilled Cheese Sandwich

Ingredients:
- 2 slices of white or whole wheat bread
- 2 slices of cheddar cheese
- 2 tablespoons unsalted butter

Equipment:
- Skillet or griddle
- Spatula

PreparationTime: 5 minutes
Cook Time: 10 minutes
Total Time: 15 minutes
Serves: 1

Directions:

1. Heat a skillet or griddle over medium heat.

2. Butter one side of each slice of bread.

3. Place one slice of bread, butter-side down, in the heated skillet.

4. Top with the two slices of cheddar cheese.

5. Place the other slice of bread, butter-side up, on top of the cheese.

6. Cook the sandwich for 3-4 minutes, or until the bottom slice is golden brown.

7. Flip the sandwich and cook for another 3-4 minutes, or until the cheese is melted and the second slice is golden brown.

8. Remove the grilled cheese sandwich from the skillet and let it cool for a minute before serving.

Storage Instructions:
- Grilled cheese sandwiches are best served immediately, but any leftovers can be stored in an airtight container in the refrigerator for up to 2 days.

Tips:
- For a 9-year-old girl, you can cut the grilled cheese sandwich in half or into quarters to make it easier to eat.
- You can also try different types of cheese, such as American, Swiss, or provolone, to mix up the flavor.
- Add a small side of fresh fruit, such as apple slices or grapes, to make it a more balanced meal.

Nutrition Information:

Calories: 350 | Total Fat: 20g | Saturated Fat: 12g | Cholesterol: 50mg | Sodium: 600mg | Total Carbohydrates: 35g | Dietary Fiber: 2g | Total Sugars: 4g | Protein: 15g

Lunches (23 Recipes)

53. Tomato Soup with Crackers

Ingredients:
- 1 cup low-sodium tomato soup
- 4-5 whole grain crackers

Equipment:
- Saucepan
- Spoon
- Bowl
- Plate

PreparationTime: 5 minutes
Cook Time: 10 minutes
Total Time: 15 minutes
Serves: 1

Directions:

1. Pour the tomato soup into a small saucepan and heat it over medium heat, stirring occasionally, until it's hot and bubbly, about 5-10 minutes.

2. Carefully pour the hot soup into a bowl.

3. Arrange the whole grain crackers on a plate and serve them alongside the tomato soup.

Storage Instructions:
- Any leftover tomato soup can be stored in an airtight container in the refrigerator for up to 3 days.

Tips:
- Encourage the 9-year-old to help with the assembly of the meal, such as pouring the soup and arranging the crackers.

- Offer a variety of crackers, such as whole wheat, multigrain, or baked, to provide different textures and flavors.

- Discuss the importance of choosing low-sodium options when it comes to canned or packaged foods.

- Serve the tomato soup with a side of fresh fruit or a small salad for a more balanced meal.

Nutrition Information:
Calories: 150 | Total Fat: 2g | Saturated Fat: 0g | Cholesterol: 0mg | Sodium: 450mg | Total Carbohydrates: 28g | Dietary Fiber: 3g | Total Sugars: 10g | Protein: 5g

Lunches (23 Recipes)

54. Tuna Salad on Whole Wheat Bread

Ingredients:
- 2 (5-ounce) cans of tuna, drained
- 2 tablespoons mayonnaise
- 1 tablespoon diced celery
- 1 tablespoon diced red onion
- 1 teaspoon lemon juice
- Salt and pepper to taste
- 2 slices of whole wheat bread

Equipment:
- Bowl
- Fork
- Knife
- Cutting board

PreparationTime: 10 minutes
Cook Time: 0 minutes
Total Time: 10 minutes
Serves: 1

Directions:
1. In a bowl, combine the drained tuna, mayonnaise, diced celery, diced red onion, and lemon juice. Mix well with a fork.

2. Season the tuna salad with salt and pepper to taste.

3. Spread the tuna salad evenly on one slice of the whole wheat bread.

4. Top with the other slice of bread to create a sandwich.

Storage Instructions:
- The tuna salad can be stored in an airtight container in the refrigerator for up to 3 days.
- The assembled sandwich can be stored in the refrigerator for up to 2 days, but it's best to assemble it just before serving.

Tips:
- For a 9-year-old girl, you can cut the sandwich in half or into quarters to make it easier to eat.
- You can also serve the tuna salad on a bed of lettuce or with whole-grain crackers for a more varied meal.
- Try adding other mix-ins to the tuna salad, such as diced pickles, chopped hard-boiled egg, or a small amount of shredded cheese.
- Encourage the 9-year-old to help prepare the tuna salad, as it's a simple and kid-friendly recipe.

Nutrition Information:

Calories: 320 | Total Fat: 15g | Saturated Fat: 3g | Cholesterol: 35mg | Sodium: 550mg | Total Carbohydrates: 30g | Dietary Fiber: 5g | Total Sugars: 4g | Protein: 20g

Lunches (23 Recipes)

55. Veggie and Hummus Wrap

Ingredients:
- 1 (8-inch) whole wheat tortilla or wrap
- 2 tablespoons hummus
- 1/4 cup shredded carrots
- 1/4 cup diced cucumber
- 1/4 cup diced bell pepper
- 1 tablespoon crumbled feta cheese (optional)
- 1 tablespoon chopped fresh parsley (optional)

PreparationTime: 10 minutes
Cook Time: 0 minutes
Total Time: 10 minutes
Serves: 1

Equipment:
- Cutting board
- Knife
- Measuring cups and spoons

Directions:

1. Spread the hummus evenly over the tortilla or wrap, leaving a 1-inch border.

2. Arrange the shredded carrots, diced cucumber, and diced bell pepper in a line down the center of the wrap.

3. If using, sprinkle the crumbled feta cheese and chopped parsley over the vegetables.

4. Fold the bottom of the wrap up over the filling, then fold in the sides and continue rolling up tightly to create a wrap.

Storage Instructions:
- Wrap the veggie and hummus wrap tightly in plastic wrap or foil and store in the refrigerator for up to 2 days.

Tips:

- For a 9-year-old girl, you can cut the wrap in half or into quarters to make it easier to eat.

- Try different combinations of vegetables, such as spinach, tomatoes, or avocado.

- You can also add a small amount of ranch or other dressing to the wrap for extra flavor.

- Serve the wrap with a side of fresh fruit or a small handful of whole-grain crackers for a more complete meal.

Nutrition Information:
Calories: 220 | Total Fat: 8g | Saturated Fat: 2g | Cholesterol: 5mg | Sodium: 450mg | Total Carbohydrates: 30g | Dietary Fiber: 6g | Total Sugars: 4g | Protein: 8g

Lunches (23 Recipes)

56. Chicken Nuggets with Carrot Sticks

Ingredients:
- 4-6 chicken nuggets (homemade or store-bought)
- 1/2 cup carrot sticks
- 1 tablespoon ranch dressing or honey mustard (for dipping)

Equipment:
- Baking sheet
- Oven
- Cutting board
- Knife

PreparationTime: 15 minutes
Cook Time: 20 minutes
Total Time: 35 minutes
Serves: 1

Directions:
1. Preheat the oven to 400°F (200°C).
2. If using homemade chicken nuggets, prepare them according to the recipe instructions and place them on a baking sheet. If using store-bought, arrange the chicken nuggets on a baking sheet.
3. Bake the chicken nuggets for 15-20 minutes, or until they are golden brown and cooked through.
4. While the chicken nuggets are baking, wash and peel the carrots. Cut the carrots into sticks, about 4 inches long and 1/2 inch thick.
5. Arrange the carrot sticks on a plate or in a small bowl.
6. Once the chicken nuggets are cooked, remove them from the oven and let them cool slightly.
7. Serve the chicken nuggets and carrot sticks with the ranch dressing or honey mustard for dipping.

Storage Instructions:
- Any leftover chicken nuggets can be stored in an airtight container in the refrigerator for up to 3 days. Reheat in the oven or microwave before serving.
- Leftover carrot sticks can be stored in an airtight container in the refrigerator for up to 5 days.

Tips:
- For a 9-year-old girl, you can cut the chicken nuggets in half or into smaller pieces to make them easier to eat.
- Encourage the 9-year-old to dip the chicken nuggets and carrot sticks in the dressing or sauce, as this can make the meal more fun and engaging.
- You can also try different dipping sauces, such as barbecue or honey mustard, to add variety.
- Serve the meal with a small side of fresh fruit or a small salad for a more balanced and nutritious meal.

Nutrition Information:

Calories: 250 | Total Fat: 12g | Saturated Fat: 3g | Cholesterol: 50mg | Sodium: 550mg | Total Carbohydrates: 18g | Dietary Fiber: 4g | Total Sugars: 6g | Protein: 18g

Lunches (23 Recipes)

57. Pita Pockets with Falafel

Ingredients:
- 1 (15 oz) can chickpeas, drained and rinsed
- 2 cloves garlic, minced
- 1/4 cup chopped parsley
- 1 teaspoon ground cumin
- 1/2 teaspoon baking soda
- 1/4 teaspoon salt
- 1 tablespoon all-purpose flour
- 2 tablespoons olive oil
- 4 whole wheat pita breads, halved
- 1/2 cup diced cucumber
- 1/4 cup crumbled feta cheese (optional)
- 2 tablespoons tahini sauce (optional)

PreparationTime: 20 minutes
Cook Time: 15 minutes
Total Time: 35 minutes
Serves: 4 pita pockets

Equipment:
- Food processor or blender - Skillet - Spatula - Plate

Directions:
1. In a food processor or blender, combine the chickpeas, garlic, parsley, cumin, baking soda, and salt. Pulse until a coarse paste forms.
2. Transfer the chickpea mixture to a bowl and stir in the flour.
3. In a skillet, heat the olive oil over medium heat.
4. Scoop heaping tablespoons of the chickpea mixture and gently place them in the hot oil. Cook for 2-3 minutes per side, or until golden brown.
5. Remove the cooked falafel from the skillet and place them on a plate lined with paper towels.
6. Stuff the pita bread halves with the warm falafel, diced cucumber, and crumbled feta cheese (if using).
7. Drizzle the tahini sauce over the falafel, if desired.

Storage Instructions:
- Store any leftover falafel in an airtight container in the refrigerator for up to 3 days.

Tips:
- Encourage the 9-year-old to help with the assembly of the pita pockets, such as stuffing the pitas and adding the toppings.
- Offer a variety of toppings, such as shredded lettuce, diced tomatoes, or sliced red onion, to customize the pita pockets.
- Serve the pita pockets with a side of fresh fruit or a small salad for a balanced meal.
- Discuss the nutritional benefits of chickpeas, such as their high protein and fiber content.

Nutrition Information:
Calories: 350 | Total Fat: 15g | Saturated Fat: 3g | Cholesterol: 5mg | Sodium: 550mg | Total Carbohydrates: 42g | Dietary Fiber: 7g | Total Sugars: 3g | Protein: 13g

Lunches (23 Recipes)

58. Spinach and Feta Stuffed Peppers

Ingredients:
- 1 bell pepper, halved and seeded
- 1/2 cup cooked spinach, drained and chopped
- 2 tablespoons crumbled feta cheese
- 1 tablespoon grated Parmesan cheese
- 1 tablespoon breadcrumbs
- 1 teaspoon olive oil
- Salt and pepper to taste

PreparationTime: 15 minutes
Cook Time: 25 minutes
Total Time: 40 minutes
Serves: 1

Equipment:
- Baking sheet
- Oven
- Mixing bowl
- Spoon

Directions:
1. Preheat the oven to 375°F (190°C).
2. Place the bell pepper halves on a baking sheet.
3. In a mixing bowl, combine the cooked spinach, crumbled feta cheese, Parmesan cheese, breadcrumbs, and olive oil. Season with salt and pepper.
4. Spoon the spinach and feta mixture evenly into the bell pepper halves.
5. Bake the stuffed peppers for 20-25 minutes, or until the peppers are tender and the filling is hot and bubbly.
6. Remove the stuffed peppers from the oven and let them cool for a few minutes before serving.

Storage Instructions:
- Any leftover stuffed peppers can be stored in an airtight container in the refrigerator for up to 3 days.

Tips:
- For a 9-year-old girl, you can cut the stuffed pepper in half or into smaller pieces to make it easier to eat.
- Try using different types of bell peppers, such as red, yellow, or orange, for variety.
- You can also experiment with different fillings, such as adding diced tomatoes, olives, or herbs to the spinach and feta mixture.
- Serve the stuffed peppers with a small side of roasted potatoes or a simple salad for a more complete meal.
- Encourage the 9-year-old to help with the preparation, such as mixing the filling or stuffing the peppers, to make the recipe more engaging.

Nutrition Information:
Calories: 180 | Total Fat: 10g | Saturated Fat: 4g | Cholesterol: 20mg | Sodium: 350mg | Total Carbohydrates: 15g | Dietary Fiber: 4g | Total Sugars: 5g | Protein: 10g

Lunches (23 Recipes)

59. Cheese and Veggie Sandwich

Ingredients:
- 2 slices of whole wheat bread
- 2 slices of cheddar cheese
- 1/4 cup shredded lettuce
- 2 slices of tomato
- 2 slices of cucumber
- 1 tablespoon mayonnaise (optional)

PreparationTime: 10 minutes
Cook Time: 0 minutes
Total Time: 10 minutes
Serves: 1

Equipment:
- Cutting board
- Knife
- Plate

Directions:

1. Lay the two slices of whole wheat bread on a clean surface.

2. Place the two slices of cheddar cheese on one of the bread slices.

3. Top the cheese with the shredded lettuce, tomato slices, and cucumber slices.

4. If using, spread the mayonnaise on the other slice of bread.

5. Place the mayonnaise-side bread on top of the vegetable-filled slice to create a sandwich.

Storage Instructions:
- The sandwich can be stored in an airtight container in the refrigerator for up to 2 days.

Tips:
- For a 9-year-old girl, you can cut the sandwich in half or into quarters to make it easier to eat.
- Try using different types of cheese, such as Swiss or provolone, to add variety.
- You can also add other vegetables, such as shredded carrots or sliced bell peppers, to the sandwich.
- Serve the sandwich with a small side of fresh fruit or a handful of whole-grain crackers for a more complete meal.
- Encourage the 9-year-old to help assemble the sandwich, as it's a simple and kid-friendly recipe.

Nutrition Information:

Calories: 320 | Total Fat: 15g | Saturated Fat: 7g | Cholesterol: 30mg | Sodium: 550mg | Total Carbohydrates: 35g | Dietary Fiber: 5g | Total Sugars: 5g | Protein: 15g

Lunches (23 Recipes)

60. Lentil Soup with Breadsticks

Ingredients:
Lentil Soup:
- 1/2 cup dried brown lentils, rinsed
- 2 cups low-sodium vegetable broth
- 1/2 cup diced carrots
- 1/2 cup diced celery
- 1/4 cup diced onion
- 1 clove garlic, minced
- 1 teaspoon dried thyme
- Salt and pepper to taste

Breadsticks:
- 1 whole wheat breadstick

Equipment:
- Saucepan- Cutting board
- Knife- Spoon

PreparationTime: 15 minutes
Cook Time: 30 minutes
Total Time: 45 minutes
Serves: 1

Nutrition Information:

Calories: 280 | Total Fat: 3g | Saturated Fat: 0g | Cholesterol: 0mg | Sodium: 450mg | Total Carbohydrates: 48g | Dietary Fiber: 12g | Total Sugars: 6g | Protein: 15g

Directions:
Lentil Soup:
1. In a saucepan, combine the rinsed lentils, vegetable broth, carrots, celery, onion, and garlic.
2. Bring the mixture to a boil, then reduce the heat and simmer for 25-30 minutes, or until the lentils are tender.
3. Stir in the dried thyme and season with salt and pepper to taste.

Breadsticks:
1. Serve the lentil soup with the whole wheat breadstick on the side.

Storage Instructions:
- The lentil soup can be stored in an airtight container in the refrigerator for up to 4 days.
- The breadstick can be stored at room temperature in a bread bag or wrapped in a clean towel for up to 3 days.

Tips:
- For a 9-year-old girl, you can serve the lentil soup in a smaller bowl or cup to make it more manageable.
- You can also break the breadstick into smaller pieces to make it easier for the 9-year-old to handle.
- Encourage the 9-year-old to dip the breadstick into the lentil soup for added flavor and texture.
- Try adding other vegetables, such as spinach or diced tomatoes, to the lentil soup for more variety.
- Serve the meal with a small side of fresh fruit or a small salad for a more balanced and nutritious meal.

Lunches (23 Recipes)

61. Sushi Rolls with Veggies

Ingredients:
- 1/2 cup cooked sushi rice
- 1 nori sheet (seaweed wrap)
- 1/4 cup julienned cucumber
- 1/4 cup julienned carrot
- 1/4 cup julienned bell pepper
- 1 tablespoon toasted sesame seeds
- Soy sauce or low-sodium soy sauce, for serving

PreparationTime: 20 minutes
Cook Time: 0 minutes
Total Time: 20 minutes
Serves: 1

Equipment:
- Bamboo sushi mat
- Sharp knife
- Cutting board
- Small bowl

Directions:
1. Lay the nori sheet shiny-side down on the sushi mat.
2. Spread the cooked sushi rice evenly over the nori sheet, leaving a 1-inch border at the top.
3. Arrange the julienned cucumber, carrot, and bell pepper in a line across the center of the rice.
4. Sprinkle the toasted sesame seeds over the vegetables.
5. Using the sushi mat, carefully roll the nori sheet tightly around the filling, starting from the bottom and rolling towards the top.
6. Wet the top 1-inch border of the nori sheet with a little water to help seal the roll.
7. Slice the sushi roll into 6-8 pieces using a sharp knife.
8. Serve the sushi rolls with soy sauce or low-sodium soy sauce for dipping.

Storage Instructions:
- The sushi rolls can be stored in an airtight container in the refrigerator for up to 2 days.

Tips:
- For a 9-year-old girl, you can cut the sushi rolls into smaller pieces or bite-sized portions to make them easier to eat.
- You can also try different vegetable fillings, such as avocado, spinach, or radish.
- Encourage the 9-year-old to help with the rolling and cutting process, as it can be a fun and interactive activity.
- Serve the sushi rolls with a small side of fresh fruit or a small salad for a more balanced meal.

Nutrition Information:

Calories: 200 | Total Fat: 3g | Saturated Fat: 0g | Cholesterol: 0mg | Sodium: 350mg | Total Carbohydrates: 38g | Dietary Fiber: 3g | Total Sugars: 3g | Protein: 5g

Lunches (23 Recipes)

62. Ham and Pineapple Skewers

Ingredients:
- 4 cubes of ham, about 1-inch each
- 4 cubes of fresh pineapple, about 1-inch each
- 1 wooden skewer

Equipment:
- Cutting board
- Knife
- Small bowl (optional)

PreparationTime: 10 minutes
Cook Time: 5 minutes
Total Time: 15 minutes
Serves: 1

Directions:
1. Thread the ham and pineapple cubes onto the wooden skewer, alternating between the two.

2. If desired, you can place the skewered ham and pineapple in a small bowl to serve.

Storage Instructions:
- The ham and pineapple skewers can be stored in an airtight container in the refrigerator for up to 2 days.

Tips:
- For a 9-year-old girl, you can cut the ham and pineapple cubes into smaller pieces to make them easier to eat.

- You can also try different combinations of ingredients, such as adding cubes of cheese or cherry tomatoes to the skewers.

- Serve the skewers with a small side of ranch dressing or honey mustard for dipping.

- Encourage the 9-year-old to help assemble the skewers, as it can be a fun and interactive activity.

- Pair the ham and pineapple skewers with a small salad or a side of fresh fruit for a more balanced meal.

Nutrition Information:

Calories: 120 | Total Fat: 3g | Saturated Fat: 1g | Cholesterol: 20mg | Sodium: 450mg | Total Carbohydrates: 15g | Dietary Fiber: 2g | Total Sugars: 12g | Protein: 8g

Lunches (23 Recipes)

63. Baked Chicken Tenders

Ingredients:
- 4-6 chicken tenders
- 1/4 cup whole wheat breadcrumbs
- 1 tablespoon grated Parmesan cheese
- 1 teaspoon dried oregano
- 1/4 teaspoon garlic powder
- Salt and pepper to taste
- 1 tablespoon olive oil

Equipment:
- Baking sheet
- Oven
- Mixing bowl
- Tongs or fork

PreparationTime: 10 minutes
Cook Time: 20 minutes
Total Time: 30 minutes
Serves: 1

Nutrition Information:
Calories: 220 | Total Fat: 9g | Saturated Fat: 2g | Cholesterol: 55mg | Sodium: 350mg | Total Carbohydrates: 12g | Dietary Fiber: 2g | Total Sugars: 1g | Protein: 22g

Directions:
1. Preheat the oven to 400°F (200°C).
2. In a mixing bowl, combine the whole wheat breadcrumbs, Parmesan cheese, dried oregano, garlic powder, salt, and pepper.
3. Drizzle the olive oil over the chicken tenders and toss to coat.
4. Dredge the chicken tenders in the breadcrumb mixture, making sure to coat them evenly on all sides.
5. Place the breaded chicken tenders on a baking sheet.
6. Bake the chicken tenders for 18-20 minutes, flipping them halfway through, until they are golden brown and cooked through.
7. Remove the baked chicken tenders from the oven and let them cool for a few minutes before serving.

Storage Instructions:
- Any leftover baked chicken tenders can be stored in an airtight container in the refrigerator for up to 3 days.

Tips:
- For a 9-year-old girl, you can cut the chicken tenders into smaller pieces or strips to make them easier to eat.
- Serve the baked chicken tenders with a small side of honey mustard or ranch dressing for dipping.
- Pair the chicken tenders with a side of roasted vegetables, such as broccoli or sweet potato fries, for a more balanced meal.
- Encourage the 9-year-old to help with the breading process, as it can be a fun and engaging activity.
- You can also try different seasoning blends, such as Italian or Cajun, to add variety to the chicken tenders.

Lunches (23 Recipes)

64. Caprese Salad with Bread

Ingredients:
- 2 slices of fresh mozzarella cheese
- 2 slices of ripe tomato
- 2 tablespoons fresh basil leaves, torn
- 1 tablespoon balsamic glaze
- 1 tablespoon olive oil
- Salt and pepper to taste
- 2 slices of whole wheat bread

PreparationTime: 10 minutes
Cook Time: 0 minutes
Total Time: 10 minutes
Serves: 1

Equipment:
- Cutting board
- Knife
- Small bowl

Directions:
1. Arrange the slices of mozzarella cheese and tomato on a plate.

2. Sprinkle the torn basil leaves over the cheese and tomatoes.

3. Drizzle the balsamic glaze and olive oil over the salad.

4. Season with salt and pepper to taste.

5. Serve the Caprese salad with the two slices of whole wheat bread.

Storage Instructions:
- The Caprese salad can be stored in an airtight container in the refrigerator for up to 2 days, but it's best to assemble it just before serving.
- The bread can be stored at room temperature in a bread bag or wrapped in a clean towel for up to 3 days.

Tips:
- For a 9-year-old girl, you can cut the Caprese salad into smaller pieces or bite-sized portions to make it easier to eat.
- You can also serve the salad with a small side of grapes or apple slices for a more complete and balanced meal.
- Encourage the 9-year-old to help assemble the Caprese salad, as it's a simple and visually appealing dish.
- If the 9-year-old doesn't like balsamic glaze, you can substitute with a drizzle of honey or a sprinkle of grated Parmesan cheese.

Nutrition Information:
Calories: 280 | Total Fat: 16g | Saturated Fat: 6g | Cholesterol: 30mg | Sodium: 450mg | Total Carbohydrates: 20g | Dietary Fiber: 3g | Total Sugars: 4g | Protein: 15g

Lunches (23 Recipes)

65. Peanut Butter and Jelly Sandwich

Ingredients:
- 2 slices of whole wheat bread
- 2 tablespoons creamy peanut butter
- 2 tablespoons fruit jam or jelly

Equipment:
- Knife
- Plate

Directions:

1. Spread the peanut butter evenly on one slice of the whole wheat bread.

2. Spread the fruit jam or jelly evenly on the other slice of bread.

3. Place the two slices of bread together to create a sandwich.

Storage Instructions:
- The peanut butter and jelly sandwich can be stored in an airtight container in the refrigerator for up to 2 days.

Tips:
- For a 9-year-old girl, you can cut the sandwich in half or into quarters to make it easier to eat.

- Try using different types of bread, such as whole grain or multigrain, for variety.

- Experiment with different types of nut butters, such as almond or cashew butter, or different fruit spreads, such as apple butter or honey.

- Serve the sandwich with a small side of fresh fruit, such as apple slices or grapes, for a more balanced meal.

- Encourage the 9-year-old to help with the preparation, such as spreading the peanut butter and jelly, to make the activity more engaging.

Nutrition Information:

Calories: 320 | Total Fat: 15g | Saturated Fat: 3g | Cholesterol: 0mg | Sodium: 350mg | Total Carbohydrates: 40g | Dietary Fiber: 5g | Total Sugars: 15g | Protein: 12g

PreparationTime: 5 minutes
Cook Time: 0 minutes
Total Time: 5 minutes
Serves: 1

Lunches (23 Recipes)

66. Turkey and Avocado Wrap

Ingredients:
- 1 (8-inch) whole wheat tortilla or wrap
- 2 slices of turkey breast
- 1/4 avocado, sliced
- 2 tablespoons shredded lettuce
- 1 tablespoon plain Greek yogurt
- 1 teaspoon Dijon mustard
- Salt and pepper to taste

PreparationTime: 10 minutes
Cook Time: 0 minutes
Total Time: 10 minutes
Serves: 1

Equipment:
- Cutting board
- Knife
- Measuring spoons

Directions:
1. Lay the whole wheat tortilla or wrap on a clean surface.

2. Place the turkey slices in the center of the wrap.

3. Top the turkey with the sliced avocado, shredded lettuce, Greek yogurt, and Dijon mustard.
4. Season with salt and pepper to taste.

5. Fold the bottom of the wrap up over the filling, then fold in the sides and continue rolling up tightly to create a wrap.

Storage Instructions:
- Wrap the turkey and avocado wrap tightly in plastic wrap or foil and store in the refrigerator for up to 2 days.

Tips:
- For a 9-year-old girl, you can cut the wrap in half or into quarters to make it easier to eat.
- Try using different types of cheese, such as cheddar or Swiss, instead of the Greek yogurt.
- You can also add other vegetables, such as diced tomatoes or shredded carrots, to the wrap.
- Serve the wrap with a small side of fresh fruit or a handful of whole-grain crackers for a more complete meal.
- Encourage the 9-year-old to help assemble the wrap, as it can be a fun and interactive activity.

Nutrition Information:

Calories: 300 | Total Fat: 12g | Saturated Fat: 3g | Cholesterol: 30mg | Sodium: 550mg | Total Carbohydrates: 32g | Dietary Fiber: 6g | Total Sugars: 3g | Protein: 18g

Lunches (23 Recipes)

67. Macaroni and Cheese

Ingredients:
- 1 cup cooked whole wheat elbow macaroni
- 2 tablespoons unsalted butter
- 2 tablespoons all-purpose flour
- 1 cup low-fat milk
- 1 cup shredded cheddar cheese
- 1/4 teaspoon salt
- 1/8 teaspoon ground black pepper

PreparationTime: 10 minutes
Cook Time: 20 minutes
Total Time: 30 minutes
Serves: 1

Equipment:
- Saucepan
- Whisk
- Measuring cups and spoons
- Strainer

Directions:
1. Cook the whole wheat elbow macaroni according to the package instructions. Drain and set aside.
2. In a saucepan, melt the butter over medium heat.
3. Whisk in the all-purpose flour and cook for 1-2 minutes, stirring constantly, to create a roux.
4. Gradually whisk in the low-fat milk and continue cooking, stirring frequently, until the sauce thickens, about 5-7 minutes.
5. Remove the saucepan from the heat and stir in the shredded cheddar cheese until it is melted and the sauce is smooth.
6. Season the cheese sauce with salt and ground black pepper.
7. Add the cooked macaroni to the cheese sauce and stir to combine.

Storage Instructions:
- The macaroni and cheese can be stored in an airtight container in the refrigerator for up to 4 days.

Tips:
- For a 9-year-old girl, you can serve the macaroni and cheese in a smaller bowl or plate to make it more manageable.
- You can also try adding diced cooked chicken or broccoli florets to the macaroni and cheese for extra nutrition.
- Encourage the 9-year-old to help with the preparation, such as measuring the ingredients or stirring the cheese sauce.
- Serve the macaroni and cheese with a small side of steamed vegetables or a fresh fruit salad for a more balanced meal.

Nutrition Information:
Calories: 380 | Total Fat: 18g | Saturated Fat: 11g | Cholesterol: 55mg | Sodium: 450mg | Total Carbohydrates: 40g | Dietary Fiber: 3g | Total Sugars: 5g | Protein: 18g

Lunches (23 Recipes)

68. Veggie Burger Sliders

Ingredients:
- 2 whole wheat slider buns or dinner rolls
- 1 veggie burger patty, cooked according to package instructions
- 2 slices of tomato
- 2 leaves of lettuce, torn into smaller pieces
- 1 tablespoon ketchup or mustard (optional)

PreparationTime: 10 minutes
Cook Time: 10 minutes
Total Time: 20 minutes
Serves: 1

Equipment:
- Skillet or griddle
- Plate

Directions:
1. Cook the veggie burger patty according to the package instructions, either in a skillet or on a griddle.

2. Once the veggie burger is cooked, place it on one of the slider buns or dinner rolls.

3. Top the veggie burger with the tomato slices and torn lettuce leaves.

4. If desired, add a small amount of ketchup or mustard to the other slider bun or dinner roll.
5. Place the top bun or roll on the veggie burger to complete the slider.

Storage Instructions:
- The cooked veggie burger sliders can be stored in an airtight container in the refrigerator for up to 2 days.

Tips:
- For a 9-year-old girl, you can cut the veggie burger slider in half or into smaller pieces to make it easier to eat.
- Try using different types of veggie burger patties, such as black bean or quinoa-based, for variety.
- Encourage the 9-year-old to help assemble the sliders, such as placing the toppings or closing the sandwiches.
- Serve the veggie burger sliders with a small side of fresh fruit or a handful of baked vegetable chips for a more balanced meal.
- If the 9-year-old doesn't like tomatoes or lettuce, you can substitute with other toppings, such as shredded carrots or cucumber slices.

Nutrition Information:

Calories: 220 | Total Fat: 8g | Saturated Fat: 1g | Cholesterol: 0mg | Sodium: 450mg | Total Carbohydrates: 28g | Dietary Fiber: 5g | Total Sugars: 5g | Protein: 10g

Lunches (23 Recipes)

69. Mini Tacos

Ingredients:
- 4-6 mini taco shells or corn tortillas
- 1/4 pound ground turkey or lean ground beef
- 2 tablespoons diced onion
- 1 teaspoon taco seasoning
- 1/4 cup shredded cheddar cheese
- 2 tablespoons diced tomatoes
- 2 tablespoons shredded lettuce
- 1 tablespoon sour cream (optional)

Equipment:
- Skillet
- Cutting board
- Knife
- Plate

PreparationTime: 15 minutes
Cook Time: 10 minutes
Total Time: 25 minutes
Serves: 1

Directions:
1. In a skillet, cook the ground turkey or beef over medium heat, breaking it up with a spoon, until it's browned and cooked through, about 5-7 minutes.
2. Add the diced onion and taco seasoning to the skillet. Stir to combine and cook for an additional 2-3 minutes.
3. Spoon the seasoned ground meat into the mini taco shells or corn tortillas.
4. Top each taco with a sprinkle of shredded cheddar cheese, diced tomatoes, and shredded lettuce.
5. If desired, add a small dollop of sour cream to each taco.

Storage Instructions:
- The cooked ground meat can be stored in an airtight container in the refrigerator for up to 3 days.
- The assembled mini tacos are best served immediately, but any leftover components can be stored separately in the refrigerator for up to 2 days.

Tips:
- For a 9-year-old girl, you can serve 2-3 mini tacos as a serving.
- Try using different types of cheese, such as Monterey Jack or pepper jack, for variety.
- Encourage the 9-year-old to help with the assembly, such as adding the toppings to the tacos.
- Serve the mini tacos with a small side of diced avocado or a side salad for a more balanced meal.
- If the 9-year-old doesn't like certain toppings, you can offer them on the side or substitute with other options, such as shredded carrots or diced bell peppers.

Nutrition Information: Calories: 260 | Total Fat: 12g | Saturated Fat: 5g | Cholesterol: 55mg | Sodium: 450mg | Total Carbohydrates: 20g | Dietary Fiber: 3g | Total Sugars: 3g | Protein: 18g

Lunches (23 Recipes)

70. Spaghetti with Meatballs

<table>
<tr><td>

Ingredients:
Meatballs:
- 1/4 pound ground beef
- 1/4 pound ground pork
- 1/4 cup breadcrumbs
- 1 tablespoon grated Parmesan cheese
- 1 teaspoon dried oregano
- 1 clove garlic, minced
- 1 egg, beaten
- Salt and pepper to taste

</td><td>

PreparationTime: 20 minutes
Cook Time: 30 minutes
Total Time: 50 minutes
Serves: 1

</td></tr>
</table>

Spaghetti:
- 1 cup cooked whole wheat spaghetti
- 1/2 cup marinara sauce

Equipment:
- Mixing bowl
- Baking sheet
- Saucepan
- Strainer

Directions:
Meatballs:
1. Preheat the oven to 400°F (200°C).
2. In a mixing bowl, combine the ground beef, ground pork, breadcrumbs, Parmesan cheese, dried oregano, garlic, and beaten egg. Season with salt and pepper.
3. Roll the mixture into 1-inch meatballs and place them on a baking sheet.
4. Bake the meatballs for 20-25 minutes, or until they are cooked through and lightly browned.

Spaghetti:
1. Cook the whole wheat spaghetti according to the package instructions.
2. Drain the cooked spaghetti and return it to the saucepan.
3. Add the marinara sauce to the spaghetti and stir to combine.

Serving:
1. Place the cooked spaghetti on a plate.
2. Top the spaghetti with the baked meatballs.

Storage Instructions:
- The meatballs can be stored in an airtight container in the refrigerator for up to 3 days.
- The cooked spaghetti with marinara sauce can be stored in an airtight container in the refrigerator for up to 4 days.

Dinner (23 Recipes)

71. Chicken and Broccoli Stir-Fry

Ingredients:
- 4 ounces boneless, skinless chicken breast, cut into bite-sized pieces
- 1 cup broccoli florets
- 1 tablespoon low-sodium soy sauce
- 1 teaspoon sesame oil
- 1 teaspoon cornstarch
- 1 clove garlic, minced
- 1/4 cup cooked brown rice

PreparationTime: 15 minutes
Cook Time: 15 minutes
Total Time: 30 minutes
Serves: 1

Equipment:
- Wok or large skillet
- Cutting board
- Knife
- Measuring cups and spoons

Directions:
1. In a small bowl, combine the soy sauce, sesame oil, and cornstarch. Mix well and set aside.
2. Heat a wok or large skillet over medium-high heat. Add the chicken and stir-fry for 3-4 minutes, or until the chicken is lightly browned.
3. Add the broccoli florets and minced garlic to the wok. Stir-fry for an additional 3-4 minutes, or until the broccoli is tender-crisp.
4. Pour the soy sauce mixture into the wok and stir to coat the chicken and broccoli. Cook for 1-2 minutes, or until the sauce has thickened.
5. Serve the chicken and broccoli stir-fry over the cooked brown rice.

Storage Instructions:
- The chicken and broccoli stir-fry can be stored in an airtight container in the refrigerator for up to 3 days.

Tips:
- For a 9-year-old girl, you can cut the chicken pieces into smaller, bite-sized chunks to make them easier to eat.
- Try using different types of vegetables, such as snow peas, carrots, or bell peppers, to add variety to the stir-fry.
- Encourage the 9-year-old to help with the preparation, such as measuring the ingredients or stirring the stir-fry.
- Serve the chicken and broccoli stir-fry with a small side of fresh fruit or a simple salad for a more balanced meal.
- If the 9-year-old doesn't like broccoli, you can substitute with another vegetable they enjoy, such as cauliflower or zucchini.

Nutrition Information:
Calories: 280 | Total Fat: 8g | Saturated Fat: 1g | Cholesterol: 65mg | Sodium: 450mg | Total Carbohydrates: 25g | Dietary Fiber: 4g | Total Sugars: 3g | Protein: 25g

Dinner (23 Recipes)

72. Baked Salmon with Green Beans

Ingredients:
- 4 ounces salmon fillet
- 1 teaspoon olive oil
- 1/2 teaspoon lemon juice
- Salt and pepper to taste
- 1 cup fresh green beans, trimmed
- 1 tablespoon water

PreparationTime: 10 minutes
Cook Time: 20 minutes
Total Time: 30 minutes
Serves: 1

Equipment:
- Baking sheet
- Oven
- Saucepan

Directions:
1. Preheat the oven to 400°F (200°C).
2. Place the salmon fillet on a baking sheet. Drizzle with the olive oil and lemon juice, and season with salt and pepper.
3. Bake the salmon for 15-20 minutes, or until it flakes easily with a fork.
4. In a saucepan, combine the trimmed green beans and 1 tablespoon of water.
5. Cover the saucepan and cook the green beans over medium heat for 5-7 minutes, or until they are tender-crisp.
6. Drain any excess water from the green beans.

Serving:
1. Place the baked salmon fillet on a plate.
2. Arrange the cooked green beans alongside the salmon.

Storage Instructions:
- The baked salmon and cooked green beans can be stored separately in airtight containers in the refrigerator for up to 2 days.

Tips:
- For a 9-year-old girl, you can cut the salmon fillet into smaller pieces or flake it with a fork to make it easier to eat.
- You can also try different seasonings on the salmon, such as garlic powder, dill, or a sprinkle of Parmesan cheese.
- Encourage the 9-year-old to help with the preparation, such as rinsing the green beans or drizzling the oil and lemon juice on the salmon.
- Serve the meal with a small side of whole grain bread or a small salad for a more complete and balanced meal.

Nutrition Information:
Calories: 250 | Total Fat: 12g | Saturated Fat: 2g | Cholesterol: 60mg | Sodium: 250mg | Total Carbohydrates: 10g | Dietary Fiber: 4g | Total Sugars: 3g | Protein: 25g

Dinner (23 Recipes)

73. Veggie Lasagna

Ingredients:
- 3 lasagna noodles, cooked according to package instructions
- 1/2 cup ricotta cheese
- 1/4 cup shredded mozzarella cheese
- 1 tablespoon grated Parmesan cheese
- 1/2 cup diced zucchini
- 1/2 cup diced bell pepper
- 1/4 cup diced onion
- 1 clove garlic, minced
- 1 cup marinara sauce
- Salt and pepper to taste

PreparationTime: 20 minutes
Cook Time: 45 minutes
Total Time: 1 hour 5 minutes
Serves: 1

Equipment: - Baking dish - Oven - Mixing bowl - Spoon

Directions:
1. Preheat the oven to 375°F (190°C).
2. In a mixing bowl, combine the ricotta cheese, 2 tablespoons of the mozzarella cheese, and the Parmesan cheese. Mix well and set aside.
3. In a separate bowl, mix the diced zucchini, bell pepper, onion, and minced garlic.
4. Spread 1/2 cup of the marinara sauce in the bottom of a baking dish.
5. Layer 3 cooked lasagna noodles over the sauce.
6. Spread the ricotta cheese mixture over the noodles.
7. Top the ricotta layer with the diced vegetable mixture.
8. Pour the remaining 1/2 cup of marinara sauce over the vegetables.
9. Sprinkle the remaining 2 tablespoons of mozzarella cheese over the top.
10. Bake the lasagna for 45 minutes, or until the cheese is melted and bubbly.
11. Remove the lasagna from the oven and let it cool for 5-10 minutes before serving.

Storage Instructions:
- The baked veggie lasagna can be stored in an airtight container in the refrigerator for up to 3 days.

Tips:
- For a 9-year-old girl, you can serve a smaller portion of the lasagna, such as a half or quarter slice.
- Try using different types of vegetables, such as spinach, mushrooms, or eggplant, to add variety.
- Encourage the 9-year-old to help with the preparation, such as layering the noodles or mixing the ricotta cheese mixture.
- Serve the veggie lasagna with a small side salad or steamed broccoli for a more balanced meal.

Nutrition Information:
Calories: 320 | Total Fat: 12g | Saturated Fat: 6g | Cholesterol: 30mg | Sodium: 550mg | Total Carbohydrates: 35g | Dietary Fiber: 4g | Total Sugars: 6g | Protein: 18g

Dinner (23 Recipes)

74. Beef Tacos with Avocado

Ingredients:
- 2 small whole wheat taco shells or corn tortillas
- 2 ounces lean ground beef
- 1 tablespoon diced onion
- 1 teaspoon taco seasoning
- 1/4 cup shredded lettuce
- 2 tablespoons diced tomatoes
- 2 tablespoons diced avocado
- 1 tablespoon shredded cheddar cheese
- 1 tablespoon plain Greek yogurt (optional)

PreparationTime: 15 minutes
Cook Time: 10 minutes
Total Time: 25 minutes
Serves: 1

Equipment:
- Skillet - Cutting board - Knife - Plate

Directions:
1. In a skillet, cook the lean ground beef over medium heat, breaking it up with a spoon, until it's browned and cooked through, about 5-7 minutes.
2. Add the diced onion and taco seasoning to the skillet. Stir to combine and cook for an additional 2-3 minutes.
3. Warm the taco shells or corn tortillas according to the package instructions.
4. Place the seasoned ground beef into the taco shells or tortillas.
5. Top each taco with the shredded lettuce, diced tomatoes, diced avocado, and shredded cheddar cheese.
6. If desired, add a small dollop of plain Greek yogurt to each taco.

Storage Instructions:
- The cooked ground beef can be stored in an airtight container in the refrigerator for up to 3 days.
- The assembled tacos are best served immediately, but any leftover components can be stored separately in the refrigerator for up to 2 days.

Tips:
- For a 9-year-old girl, you can serve 1-2 small tacos as a serving.
- Try using different types of cheese, such as Monterey Jack or pepper jack, for variety.
- Encourage the 9-year-old to help with the assembly, such as adding the toppings to the tacos.
- Serve the beef tacos with a small side of diced mango or a small salad for a more balanced meal.
- If the 9-year-old doesn't like certain toppings, you can offer them on the side or substitute with other options, such as shredded carrots or diced bell peppers.

Nutrition Information: Calories: 280 | Total Fat: 13g | Saturated Fat: 5g | Cholesterol: 50mg | Sodium: 450mg | Total Carbohydrates: 22g | Dietary Fiber: 5g | Total Sugars: 3g | Protein: 20g

Dinner (23 Recipes)

75. Chicken Alfredo Pasta

Ingredients:
- 1 cup cooked whole wheat pasta
- 2 ounces grilled or baked chicken breast, diced
- 2 tablespoons low-fat Alfredo sauce
- 1 tablespoon grated Parmesan cheese
- 1 tablespoon frozen peas (optional)
- Salt and pepper to taste

Equipment:
- Saucepan
- Strainer
- Cutting board
- Knife

PreparationTime: 15 minutes
Cook Time: 20 minutes
Total Time: 35 minutes
Serves: 1

Directions:
1. Cook the whole wheat pasta according to the package instructions. Drain and set aside.
2. In a saucepan, warm the low-fat Alfredo sauce over medium heat, stirring occasionally, until heated through.
3. Add the cooked pasta and diced chicken to the Alfredo sauce. Stir to combine.
4. If using, add the frozen peas and stir until they are heated through.
5. Remove the pasta from the heat and sprinkle the grated Parmesan cheese on top.
6. Season with salt and pepper to taste.

Storage Instructions:
- The chicken Alfredo pasta can be stored in an airtight container in the refrigerator for up to 3 days.

Tips:
- For a 9-year-old girl, you can serve the pasta in a smaller bowl or plate to make it more manageable.
- Try using a whole wheat pasta with a fun shape, such as spirals or bow ties, to make it more appealing.
- You can also add other vegetables, such as broccoli or diced tomatoes, to the pasta for extra nutrition.
- Encourage the 9-year-old to help with the preparation, such as measuring the ingredients or stirring the pasta.
- Serve the chicken Alfredo pasta with a small side of steamed vegetables or a fresh fruit salad for a more balanced meal.

Nutrition Information:
Calories: 380 | Total Fat: 12g | Saturated Fat: 5g | Cholesterol: 55mg | Sodium: 450mg | Total Carbohydrates: 45g | Dietary Fiber: 5g | Total Sugars: 3g | Protein: 25g

Dinner (23 Recipes)

76. Baked Ziti with Ricotta

Ingredients:
- 1 lb ziti pasta
- 1 lb ground beef or Italian sausage
- 1 onion, diced
- 3 cloves garlic, minced
- 1 (24 oz) jar marinara sauce
- 1 (15 oz) container ricotta cheese
- 2 cups shredded mozzarella cheese
- 1/2 cup grated Parmesan cheese
- 2 eggs
- 1/4 cup chopped fresh parsley
- Salt and pepper to taste

PreparationTime: 20 minutes
Cook Time: 45 minutes
Total Time: 1 hour 5 minutes
Serves: 6-8

Equipment:
- Large pot
- Skillet
- Mixing bowl
- 9x13 inch baking dish

Directions:
1. Preheat oven to 375°F.
2. Bring a large pot of salted water to a boil. Cook the ziti according to package instructions until al dente. Drain and set aside.
3. In a skillet, cook the ground beef or sausage over medium heat until browned and crumbled. Drain excess fat.
4. Add the onion and garlic to the skillet and cook for 2-3 minutes until softened.
5. Stir in the marinara sauce and simmer for 5 minutes.
6. In a mixing bowl, combine the ricotta cheese, 1 cup of the mozzarella cheese, Parmesan cheese, eggs, and parsley. Season with salt and pepper.
7. Spread a thin layer of the meat sauce in the bottom of the baking dish. Layer half of the cooked ziti, then top with half of the ricotta mixture and half of the remaining meat sauce. Repeat the layers.
8. Top with the remaining 1 cup of mozzarella cheese.
9. Bake for 45 minutes, or until the cheese is melted and bubbly.
10. Let stand for 5-10 minutes before serving.

Storage Instructions:
Leftovers can be stored in an airtight container in the refrigerator for up to 4 days. Reheat in the oven or microwave before serving.

Tips:
- Use a combination of ground beef and Italian sausage for more flavor.
- Adjust the amount of ricotta and mozzarella cheese to your liking.
- Garnish with fresh basil or parsley before serving.

Dinner (23 Recipes)

77. Grilled Chicken with Quinoa

Ingredients:
- 4 boneless, skinless chicken breasts
- 1 cup quinoa, rinsed
- 2 cups low-sodium chicken broth
- 1 cup diced bell peppers (any color)
- 1 cup diced cucumber
- 1/2 cup diced red onion
- 2 tbsp chopped fresh parsley
- 2 tbsp olive oil
- 2 tbsp lemon juice
- 1 tsp garlic powder
- Salt and pepper to taste

PreparationTime: 15 minutes
Cook Time: 30 minutes
Total Time: 45 minutes
Serves: 4

Equipment: - Grill or grill pan - Saucepan - Mixing bowl

Directions:
1. Preheat your grill or grill pan to medium-high heat.
2. In a saucepan, combine the quinoa and chicken broth. Bring to a boil, then reduce heat to low, cover, and simmer for 15-20 minutes, or until the quinoa is tender and the liquid is absorbed.
3. While the quinoa is cooking, season the chicken breasts with garlic powder, salt, and pepper.
4. Grill the chicken for 5-7 minutes per side, or until it's cooked through and reaches an internal temperature of 165°F.
5. In a mixing bowl, combine the cooked quinoa, diced bell peppers, cucumber, red onion, and parsley.
6. Drizzle the olive oil and lemon juice over the quinoa mixture and toss to coat.
7. Serve the grilled chicken on top of the quinoa salad.

Storage Instructions:
Leftover grilled chicken and quinoa can be stored in an airtight container in the refrigerator for up to 3 days. Reheat the chicken and quinoa separately before serving.

Tips:
- Encourage your 9-year-old to help with the preparation, such as rinsing the quinoa or mixing the quinoa salad.
- Offer a variety of colorful vegetables to make the dish more appealing to your child.
- Adjust the seasoning to your child's taste preferences.
- Serve the dish with a side of fresh fruit or a small salad for a well-rounded meal.

Nutrition Information:
This grilled chicken and quinoa dish provides a balanced and nutritious meal for a 9-year-old girl. The chicken is a lean source of protein, while the quinoa is a whole grain that provides complex carbohydrates, fiber, and essential vitamins and minerals. The vegetables add additional nutrients and fiber, making this a well-rounded and satisfying meal.

Dinner (23 Recipes)

78. Shepherd's Pie

Ingredients:
- 1 lb ground lamb (or ground beef)
- 1 onion, diced
- 2 carrots, peeled and diced
- 2 celery stalks, diced
- 2 cloves garlic, minced
- 2 tablespoons tomato paste
- 1 cup beef or chicken stock
- 2 tablespoons Worcestershire sauce
- 1 teaspoon dried thyme
- Salt and pepper to taste
- 3 lbs russet potatoes, peeled and cut into 1-inch cubes
- 4 tablespoons unsalted butter
- 1/2 cup milk
- 1 cup shredded cheddar cheese

PreparationTime: 20 minutes
Cook Time: 45 minutes
Total Time: 1 hour 5 minutes
Serves: 4-6

Equipment: - Large skillet or Dutch oven - Potato masher or ricer - Baking dish (9x13 inch)

Directions:
1. Preheat oven to 375°F.
2. In a large skillet or Dutch oven, cook the ground lamb over medium-high heat until browned and crumbled, 5-7 minutes. Drain any excess fat.
3. Add the onion, carrots, celery, and garlic to the skillet. Cook for 5-7 minutes, until the vegetables are softened.
4. Stir in the tomato paste and cook for 1 minute.
5. Add the stock, Worcestershire sauce, and thyme. Bring to a simmer and cook for 10-15 minutes, until the sauce has thickened.
6. Season with salt and pepper to taste.
7. Meanwhile, in a large pot, cover the potato cubes with cold water. Bring to a boil and cook until tender, 15-20 minutes. Drain and return to the pot.
8. Add the butter and milk to the potatoes and mash until smooth and creamy.
9. Spread the lamb mixture into a 9x13 inch baking dish. Top with the mashed potatoes and sprinkle with the cheddar cheese.
10. Bake for 25-30 minutes, until the potatoes are lightly browned and the filling is bubbling.
11. Let stand for 5 minutes before serving.

Storage Instructions:
Leftover shepherd's pie can be stored in an airtight container in the refrigerator for up to 3 days. Reheat in the oven or microwave before serving.

Nutrition Information:
Calories: 550 | Protein: 30g | Carbohydrates: 50g | Fat: 27g | Saturated Fat: 14g | Cholesterol: 100mg | Sodium: 650mg | Fiber: 5g | Sugar: 5g

Dinner (23 Recipes)

79. Veggie and Cheese Pizza

Ingredients:
- 1 pre-made pizza crust or dough
- 1 cup marinara or pizza sauce
- 1 cup shredded mozzarella cheese
- 1/2 cup grated Parmesan cheese
- 1 cup sliced mushrooms
- 1 cup diced bell peppers (any color)
- 1 cup diced onions
- 1 cup cherry tomatoes, halved
- 1/4 cup sliced black olives (optional)
- 1 tsp dried oregano
- Salt and pepper to taste

PreparationTime: 20 minutes
Cook Time: 15-20 minutes
Total Time: 35-40 minutes
Serves: 4-6

Equipment:
- Baking sheet or pizza pan
- Cutting board and knife
- Mixing bowl

Directions:
1. Preheat your oven to 400°F.
2. If using pre-made dough, roll or stretch it out to fit your baking sheet or pizza pan. If using a pre-made crust, skip this step.
3. Spread the marinara or pizza sauce evenly over the crust.
4. Sprinkle the mozzarella and Parmesan cheeses over the sauce.
5. Arrange the sliced mushrooms, diced bell peppers, onions, and cherry tomatoes over the cheese.
6. If using, sprinkle the sliced black olives over the top.
7. Sprinkle the dried oregano and season with salt and pepper to taste.
8. Bake the pizza for 15-20 minutes, or until the crust is golden brown and the cheese is melted and bubbly.
9. Let the pizza cool for a few minutes before slicing and serving.

Storage Instructions:
Leftover pizza can be stored in an airtight container in the refrigerator for up to 3 days. Reheat in the oven or microwave before serving.

Tips:
- Encourage your 9-year-old to help with the preparation, such as spreading the sauce or arranging the toppings.
- Offer a variety of vegetable toppings to encourage your child to try new things.
- Serve the pizza with a side salad or fresh fruit for a well-rounded meal.
- Adjust the toppings to your child's preferences, such as adding or removing certain vegetables.

Dinner (23 Recipes)

80. Shrimp Fried Rice

Ingredients:
- 1 lb shrimp, peeled and deveined
- 2 cups cooked white rice, chilled
- 2 tablespoons vegetable oil
- 2 cloves garlic, minced
- 1 onion, diced
- 1 cup frozen peas and carrots
- 2 eggs, beaten
- 2 tablespoons soy sauce
- 1 teaspoon sesame oil
- Salt and pepper to taste

PreparationTime: 15 minutes
Cook Time: 15 minutes
Total Time: 30 minutes
Serves: 4

Equipment:
- Wok or large skillet
- Spatula
- Cutting board and knife

Directions:
1. Heat the vegetable oil in a wok or large skillet over high heat.
2. Add the shrimp and cook for 2-3 minutes, until they start to turn pink. Remove the shrimp from the wok and set aside.
3. Add the garlic and onion to the wok and cook for 2-3 minutes, until fragrant and translucent.
4. Add the cooked rice and frozen peas and carrots to the wok. Stir-fry for 3-4 minutes, breaking up any clumps of rice.
5. Push the rice mixture to the side of the wok and pour the beaten eggs into the empty space. Scramble the eggs for 1-2 minutes, then mix them into the rice.
6. Add the cooked shrimp, soy sauce, and sesame oil to the wok. Stir-fry for 2-3 minutes, until everything is heated through.
7. Season with salt and pepper to taste.

Storage Instructions:
Leftover shrimp fried rice can be stored in an airtight container in the refrigerator for up to 3 days.

Tips:
- Use day-old rice for best results, as it will be drier and less likely to clump.
- Adjust the amount of soy sauce and sesame oil to your taste.
- Add any other vegetables you like, such as bell peppers or mushrooms.

Nutrition Information:
Calories: 300 | Protein: 22g | Carbohydrates: 30g | Fat: 10g | Saturated Fat: 2g | Cholesterol: 170mg | Sodium: 800mg | Fiber: 3g | Sugar: 3g

Dinner (23 Recipes)

81. Stuffed Bell Peppers

Ingredients:
- 4-6 bell peppers (any color)
- 1 lb ground turkey or lean ground beef
- 1 cup cooked rice
- 1 small onion, diced
- 2 cloves garlic, minced
- 1 (15 oz) can diced tomatoes
- 1/2 cup shredded mozzarella cheese
- 1/4 cup grated Parmesan cheese
- 1 tsp dried oregano
- Salt and pepper to taste

Equipment: - Large pot - Skillet - Mixing bowl - 9x13 inch baking dish

PreparationTime: 20 minutes
Cook Time: 45 minutes
Total Time: 1 hour 5 minutes
Serves: 4-6

Directions:
1. Preheat oven to 375°F.
2. Cut the tops off the bell peppers and remove the seeds and membranes. Place the peppers in a large pot and cover with water. Bring to a boil and parboil for 5 minutes. Drain and set aside.
3. In a skillet, cook the ground turkey or beef over medium heat until browned and crumbled. Drain excess fat.
4. Add the onion and garlic to the skillet and cook for 2-3 minutes until softened.
5. Stir in the diced tomatoes, cooked rice, oregano, salt, and pepper. Mix well.
6. Stuff the parboiled bell peppers with the meat and rice mixture, packing it in tightly.
7. Place the stuffed peppers in the baking dish and top with the mozzarella and Parmesan cheeses.
8. Bake for 45 minutes, or until the peppers are tender and the cheese is melted and bubbly.
9. Let stand for 5-10 minutes before serving.

Storage Instructions:
Leftovers can be stored in an airtight container in the refrigerator for up to 3 days. Reheat in the oven or microwave before serving.

Tips:
- Use a combination of ground turkey and ground beef for more flavor.
- Adjust the amount of cheese to your child's preference.
- Serve with a side of steamed vegetables or a fresh salad for a well-rounded meal.

Nutrition Information:
This recipe provides a balanced and nutritious meal for a 9-year-old girl, with a good source of protein, carbohydrates, and essential vitamins and minerals. The bell peppers are a great source of vitamin C, while the ground turkey or beef provides lean protein. The rice and cheese add additional nutrients and flavor.

Dinner (23 Recipes)

82. BBQ Chicken Drumsticks

Ingredients:
- 8 chicken drumsticks
- 1/2 cup barbecue sauce
- 1 tablespoon honey
- 1 teaspoon garlic powder
- 1/2 teaspoon smoked paprika
- 1/4 teaspoon salt
- 1/4 teaspoon black pepper

PreparationTime: 10 minutes
Cook Time: 40 minutes
Total Time: 50 minutes
Serves: 4

Equipment:
- Baking sheet or shallow baking dish
- Mixing bowl
- Tongs or spoon

Directions:
1. Preheat your oven to 400°F.
2. In a mixing bowl, combine the barbecue sauce, honey, garlic powder, smoked paprika, salt, and black pepper. Whisk the ingredients together until well mixed.
3. Place the chicken drumsticks on a baking sheet or in a shallow baking dish. Brush the drumsticks with the barbecue sauce mixture, making sure to coat them evenly.
4. Bake the drumsticks in the preheated oven for 40-45 minutes, turning and basting them with the sauce halfway through the cooking time.
5. Once the drumsticks are cooked through and the sauce is caramelized, remove them from the oven.
6. Serve the BBQ chicken drumsticks warm, with any extra sauce drizzled over the top.

Storage Instructions:
Leftover BBQ chicken drumsticks can be stored in an airtight container in the refrigerator for up to 3 days. Reheat in the oven or microwave before serving.

Tips:
- Encourage your 9-year-old to help with the preparation, such as brushing the drumsticks with the sauce.
- Serve the drumsticks with a side of roasted vegetables or a fresh salad for a balanced meal.
- For a fun presentation, you can serve the drumsticks with small bowls of extra barbecue sauce for dipping.

Nutrition Information:
Calories: 280 | Protein: 26g | Carbohydrates: 16g | Fat: 13g | Saturated Fat: 3.5g | Cholesterol: 135mg | Sodium: 650mg | Fiber: 0g | Sugar: 14g

Dinner (23 Recipes)

83. Veggie Frittata

Ingredients:
- 6 eggs
- 1/4 cup milk
- 1/2 teaspoon salt
- 1/4 teaspoon black pepper
- 1 tablespoon olive oil
- 1 cup diced bell peppers (any color)
- 1 cup diced zucchini
- 1/2 cup diced onion
- 1 cup baby spinach leaves
- 1/2 cup shredded cheddar cheese

PreparationTime: 15 minutes
Cook Time: 25 minutes
Total Time: 40 minutes
Serves: 4

Equipment:
- 9-inch oven-safe skillet or pie dish
- Whisk
- Cutting board and knife

Directions:
1. Preheat your oven to 375°F.
2. In a medium bowl, whisk together the eggs, milk, salt, and pepper until well combined.
3. Heat the olive oil in the oven-safe skillet over medium heat.
4. Add the diced bell peppers, zucchini, and onion to the skillet. Cook for 5-7 minutes, stirring occasionally, until the vegetables are tender.
5. Add the baby spinach leaves to the skillet and cook for 1-2 minutes, until the spinach is wilted.
6. Pour the egg mixture over the vegetables in the skillet. Sprinkle the shredded cheddar cheese on top.
7. Transfer the skillet to the preheated oven and bake for 18-22 minutes, or until the frittata is set and the cheese is melted and bubbly.
8. Remove the frittata from the oven and let it cool for 5 minutes before slicing and serving.

Storage Instructions:
Leftover veggie frittata can be stored in an airtight container in the refrigerator for up to 3 days. Reheat slices in the microwave or oven before serving.

Tips:
- Encourage your 9-year-old to help with the preparation, such as whisking the eggs or sprinkling the cheese.
- Adjust the vegetable ingredients to your child's preferences, such as using their favorite veggies.
- Serve the frittata with a side of fresh fruit or a small salad for a balanced meal.

Nutrition Information:
Calories: 220 | Protein: 16g | Carbohydrates: 8g | Fat: 14g | Saturated Fat: 6g | Cholesterol: 260mg | Sodium: 480mg | Fiber: 2g | Sugar: 4g

Dinner (23 Recipes)

84. Baked Tilapia with Lemon

Ingredients:
- 4 tilapia fillets (about 1 lb total)
- 2 tablespoons olive oil
- 2 tablespoons lemon juice
- 1 teaspoon grated lemon zest
- 1 teaspoon dried parsley
- 1/2 teaspoon garlic powder
- 1/4 teaspoon salt
- 1/4 teaspoon black pepper

PreparationTime: 10 minutes
Cook Time: 20 minutes
Total Time: 30 minutes
Serves: 4

Equipment:
- Baking sheet or oven-safe dish
- Parchment paper or foil
- Zester or grater

Directions:
1. Preheat your oven to 400°F.
2. Line a baking sheet or oven-safe dish with parchment paper or foil.
3. Place the tilapia fillets on the prepared baking sheet or dish.
4. In a small bowl, whisk together the olive oil, lemon juice, lemon zest, dried parsley, garlic powder, salt, and black pepper.
5. Drizzle the lemon-herb mixture over the tilapia fillets, making sure to evenly coat the fish.
6. Bake the tilapia in the preheated oven for 18-22 minutes, or until the fish flakes easily with a fork and is opaque throughout.
7. Serve the baked tilapia with lemon wedges, if desired.

Storage Instructions:
Leftover baked tilapia can be stored in an airtight container in the refrigerator for up to 3 days. Reheat in the oven or microwave before serving.

Tips:
- Encourage your child to help with the preparation, such as measuring the ingredients or drizzling the lemon-herb mixture over the fish.
- Serve the baked tilapia with a side of roasted vegetables or a fresh salad for a balanced meal.
- Experiment with different herbs and spices to find your child's favorite flavor combination.
- If your child doesn't like tilapia, you can substitute another mild white fish, such as cod or halibut.

Nutrition Information:
Calories: 180 | Protein: 27g | Carbohydrates: 2g | Fat: 8g | Saturated Fat: 1g | Cholesterol: 55mg | Sodium: 300mg | Fiber: 0g | Sugar: 0g

Dinner (23 Recipes)

85. Chicken and Veggie Skewers

Ingredients:
- 1 lb boneless, skinless chicken breasts, cut into 1-inch cubes
- 1 red bell pepper, cut into 1-inch pieces
- 1 yellow bell pepper, cut into 1-inch pieces
- 1 zucchini, cut into 1-inch slices
- 1 red onion, cut into 1-inch pieces
- 2 tablespoons olive oil
- 1 teaspoon dried oregano
- 1/2 teaspoon garlic powder
- 1/4 teaspoon salt
- 1/4 teaspoon black pepper

PreparationTime: 20 minutes
Cook Time: 15 minutes
Total Time: 35 minutes
Serves: 4

Equipment:
- Wooden or metal skewers - Baking sheet or grill

Directions:
1. Preheat your oven to 400°F or prepare your grill for medium-high heat.
2. In a large bowl, combine the cubed chicken, bell pepper pieces, zucchini slices, and red onion pieces.
3. Drizzle the olive oil over the chicken and vegetables, and then sprinkle the oregano, garlic powder, salt, and black pepper over the top. Toss everything together until the chicken and vegetables are evenly coated.
4. Thread the chicken and vegetables onto the skewers, alternating the ingredients.
5. If baking, place the skewers on a baking sheet and bake for 15-18 minutes, turning halfway, until the chicken is cooked through and the vegetables are tender.
6. If grilling, place the skewers directly on the grill grates and cook for 12-15 minutes, turning occasionally, until the chicken is cooked through and the vegetables are tender.
7. Serve the chicken and veggie skewers warm, with any desired dipping sauces or toppings.

Storage Instructions:
Leftover chicken and veggie skewers can be stored in an airtight container in the refrigerator for up to 3 days. Reheat in the oven or on the grill before serving.

Tips:
- Encourage your 9-year-old to help with the preparation, such as threading the ingredients onto the skewers.
- Offer a variety of dipping sauces, like ranch, barbecue, or honey mustard, for your child to enjoy.
- Serve the skewers with a side of roasted potatoes or a fresh salad for a balanced meal.
- Adjust the vegetable selection to include your child's favorite veggies.

Nutrition Information:
Calories: 250 | Protein: 25g | Carbohydrates: 12g | Fat: 11g | Saturated Fat: 2g | Cholesterol: 70mg | Sodium: 300mg | Fiber: 3g | Sugar: 6g

Dinner (23 Recipes)

86. Beef and Bean Chili

Ingredients:
- 1 lb ground beef
- 1 onion, diced
- 2 cloves garlic, minced
- 1 tablespoon chili powder
- 1 teaspoon ground cumin
- 1 teaspoon dried oregano
- 1/2 teaspoon salt
- 1/4 teaspoon black pepper
- 1 (15 oz) can diced tomatoes
- 1 (15 oz) can kidney beans, drained and rinsed
- 1 (15 oz) can black beans, drained and rinsed
- 1 cup beef broth

PreparationTime: 15 minutes
Cook Time: 45 minutes
Total Time: 1 hour
Serves: 4

Equipment:
- Large pot or Dutch oven - Wooden spoon - Can opener

Directions:
1. In a large pot or Dutch oven, cook the ground beef over medium-high heat until browned and crumbled, about 5-7 minutes. Drain any excess fat.
2. Add the diced onion and minced garlic to the pot. Cook for 2-3 minutes, until the onion is translucent.
3. Stir in the chili powder, cumin, oregano, salt, and black pepper. Cook for 1 minute to toast the spices.
4. Add the diced tomatoes, kidney beans, black beans, and beef broth to the pot. Stir to combine.
5. Bring the chili to a simmer and let it cook for 30-40 minutes, stirring occasionally, until the flavors have melded and the chili has thickened.
6. Taste and adjust the seasoning as needed.
7. Serve the beef and bean chili hot, with optional toppings like shredded cheese, sour cream, or chopped green onions.

Storage Instructions:
Leftover chili can be stored in an airtight container in the refrigerator for up to 4 days. It can also be frozen for up to 3 months.

Tips:
- Encourage your 9-year-old to help with the preparation, such as measuring the spices or stirring the chili.
- Serve the chili with cornbread or tortilla chips for dipping.
- Adjust the spice level to your child's preference by using less chili powder or adding a milder chili powder.
- Top the chili with your child's favorite toppings, like shredded cheese or crushed tortilla chips.

Dinner (23 Recipes)

87. Veggie Stir-Fry with Tofu

Ingredients:
- 1 block (14 oz) firm or extra-firm tofu, cubed
- 2 tablespoons vegetable oil
- 1 cup broccoli florets
- 1 cup sliced carrots
- 1 cup snow peas or snap peas
- 1 red bell pepper, sliced
- 1 cup sliced mushrooms
- 2 cloves garlic, minced
- 2 tablespoons low-sodium soy sauce
- 1 tablespoon honey
- 1 teaspoon sesame oil
- Salt and pepper to taste
- Cooked brown rice, for serving

Equipment:
- Wok or large skillet
- Cutting board and knife
- Spatula or tongs

PreparationTime: 15 minutes
Cook Time: 15 minutes
Total Time: 30 minutes
Serves: 4

Nutrition Information:
Calories: 280 | Protein: 18g | Carbohydrates: 25g | Fat: 13g | Saturated Fat: 2g | Cholesterol: 0mg | Sodium: 450mg | Fiber: 5g | Sugar: 8g

Directions:
1. Press the tofu block between paper towels or a clean kitchen towel to remove excess moisture. Cut the tofu into 1-inch cubes.
2. Heat the vegetable oil in a wok or large skillet over high heat.
3. Add the tofu cubes and cook, stirring occasionally, until lightly browned on all sides, about 5-7 minutes. Remove the tofu from the wok and set aside.
4. Add the broccoli, carrots, snow peas, bell pepper, and mushrooms to the wok. Stir-fry for 5-7 minutes, until the vegetables are tender-crisp.
5. Add the garlic to the wok and cook for 1 minute, until fragrant.
6. In a small bowl, whisk together the soy sauce, honey, and sesame oil.
7. Add the cooked tofu back to the wok and pour the soy sauce mixture over the top. Toss everything together and cook for 2-3 minutes, until the sauce has thickened slightly.
8. Season with salt and pepper to taste.
9. Serve the veggie stir-fry with tofu over a bed of cooked brown rice.

Storage Instructions:
Leftover veggie stir-fry with tofu can be stored in an airtight container in the refrigerator for up to 3 days. Reheat in the microwave or on the stove before serving.

Tips:
- Encourage your 9-year-old to help with the preparation, such as measuring the ingredients or stirring the stir-fry.
- Adjust the vegetables to include your child's favorites, such as broccoli, carrots, and bell peppers.

Dinner (23 Recipes)

88. Grilled Cheese and Tomato Soup

Ingredients:
Grilled Cheese:
- 2 slices of bread
- 2 slices of cheddar cheese
- 2 teaspoons butter

Tomato Soup:
- 1 cup canned tomato soup
- 1/4 cup milk

Equipment:
- Skillet or griddle
- Spatula
- Small saucepan

Directions:
Grilled Cheese:
1. Heat a skillet or griddle over medium heat.
2. Butter one side of each slice of bread.
3. Place one slice of bread, butter-side down, in the skillet. Top with the cheddar cheese slices, then the other slice of bread, butter-side up.
4. Cook the grilled cheese for 2-3 minutes per side, or until the bread is golden brown and the cheese is melted.
5. Remove the grilled cheese from the skillet and cut it in half.

Tomato Soup:
1. In a small saucepan, combine the canned tomato soup and milk.
2. Heat the soup over medium heat, stirring occasionally, until it's hot and bubbly.

Serving:
1. Serve the grilled cheese sandwich and the hot tomato soup together, with the grilled cheese cut in half to make it easier for your 9-year-old to dip and enjoy.

Storage Instructions:
Leftover grilled cheese and tomato soup can be stored separately in airtight containers in the refrigerator for up to 3 days. Reheat the soup on the stove or in the microwave, and the grilled cheese in a skillet or toaster oven before serving.

Nutrition Information:
Grilled Cheese:
Calories: 350 | Protein: 16g | Carbohydrates: 32g | Fat: 19g | Saturated Fat: 11g | Cholesterol: 50mg | Sodium: 680mg | Fiber: 2g | Sugar: 4g

Dinner (23 Recipes)

89. Chicken Pot Pie

Ingredients:
- 1 lb boneless, skinless chicken breasts, cubed
- 2 tablespoons olive oil
- 1 onion, diced
- 2 carrots, peeled and diced
- 2 celery stalks, diced
- 2 cloves garlic, minced
- 2 tablespoons all-purpose flour
- 1 cup chicken broth
- 1 cup milk
- 1 teaspoon dried thyme
- 1/2 teaspoon salt
- 1/4 teaspoon black pepper
- 1 cup frozen peas
- 1 (9-inch) refrigerated pie crust

PreparationTime: 30 minutes
Cook Time: 40 minutes
Total Time: 1 hour 10 minutes
Serves: 4

Equipment:
- Large skillet or Dutch oven
- Baking dish (9-inch pie dish or 8x8 inch baking dish)
- Rolling pin

Directions:
1. Preheat your oven to 400°F.
2. In a large skillet or Dutch oven, heat the olive oil over medium-high heat. Add the cubed chicken and cook until browned, about 5-7 minutes. Remove the chicken from the skillet and set aside.
3. Add the diced onion, carrots, celery, and garlic to the skillet. Cook for 5-7 minutes, until the vegetables are softened.
4. Sprinkle the flour over the vegetables and stir to coat. Cook for 1 minute.
5. Gradually whisk in the chicken broth and milk. Bring the mixture to a simmer and cook for 5-7 minutes, until thickened.
6. Stir in the cooked chicken, dried thyme, salt, and black pepper. Add the frozen peas and stir to combine.
7. Transfer the chicken and vegetable mixture to a 9-inch pie dish or 8x8 inch baking dish.
8. Unroll the refrigerated pie crust and place it over the filling, pressing the edges to seal. Cut a few slits in the top of the crust to allow steam to escape.
9. Bake the chicken pot pie in the preheated oven for 30-35 minutes, or until the crust is golden brown and the filling is bubbling.
10. Let the pot pie cool for 5-10 minutes before serving.

Storage Instructions:
Leftover chicken pot pie can be stored in an airtight container in the refrigerator for up to 3 days. Reheat in the oven or microwave before serving.

Dinner (23 Recipes)

90. Pork Chops with Mashed Potatoes

Ingredients:
Pork Chops:
- 4 boneless pork chops (about 1 lb total)
- 1 tablespoon olive oil
- 1 teaspoon garlic powder
- 1 teaspoon dried thyme
- 1/2 teaspoon salt
- 1/4 teaspoon black pepper

Mashed Potatoes:
- 3 lbs russet potatoes, peeled and cut into 1-inch cubes
- 1/2 cup milk
- 4 tablespoons unsalted butter
- 1/2 teaspoon salt
- 1/4 teaspoon black pepper

Equipment:
- Baking sheet or oven-safe skillet
- Potato masher or ricer
- Saucepan

Directions:
Pork Chops:
1. Preheat your oven to 400°F.
2. Pat the pork chops dry with paper towels and place them on a baking sheet or in an oven-safe skillet.
3. Drizzle the olive oil over the pork chops and rub it in to coat them evenly.
4. Sprinkle the garlic powder, dried thyme, salt, and black pepper over the pork chops, making sure to season both sides.
5. Bake the pork chops in the preheated oven for 20-25 minutes, or until they reach an internal temperature of 145°F.
6. Let the pork chops rest for 5 minutes before serving.

Mashed Potatoes:
1. In a large saucepan, cover the potato cubes with cold water.
2. Bring the water to a boil over high heat, then reduce the heat to medium-low and simmer for 15-20 minutes, or until the potatoes are tender when pierced with a fork.
3. Drain the potatoes and return them to the saucepan.
4. Add the milk and butter to the potatoes and mash them with a potato masher or ricer until smooth and creamy.
5. Stir in the salt and black pepper.
6. Keep the mashed potatoes warm until ready to serve.

PreparationTime: 20 minutes
Cook Time: 30 minutes
Total Time: 50 minutes
Serves: 4

Dinner (23 Recipes)

91. Veggie Enchiladas

Ingredients:
- 1 tablespoon olive oil
- 1 onion, diced
- 1 bell pepper, diced
- 1 cup sliced mushrooms
- 1 cup frozen corn kernels
- 1 (15 oz) can black beans, drained and rinsed
- 1 teaspoon chili powder
- 1/2 teaspoon cumin
- 1/4 teaspoon garlic powder
- Salt and pepper to taste
- 8 (6-inch) whole wheat tortillas
- 1 (15 oz) can enchilada sauce
- 1 cup shredded cheddar cheese

Equipment:
- Baking dish (9x13 inch)
- Skillet
- Mixing bowl
- Spoon or spatula

PreparationTime: 25 minutes
Cook Time: 30 minutes
Total Time: 55 minutes
Serves: 4

Directions:
1. Preheat your oven to 375°F.
2. In a skillet, heat the olive oil over medium heat. Add the diced onion, bell pepper, sliced mushrooms, and frozen corn. Sauté for 5-7 minutes, until the vegetables are tender.
3. Stir in the drained and rinsed black beans, chili powder, cumin, garlic powder, and a pinch of salt and pepper. Cook for 2-3 minutes, until the flavors are combined.
4. Spread about 1/4 cup of the vegetable mixture onto the center of each whole wheat tortilla. Roll up the tortillas and place them seam-side down in a 9x13 inch baking dish.
5. Pour the enchilada sauce evenly over the rolled enchiladas. Sprinkle the shredded cheddar cheese on top.
6. Bake the enchiladas in the preheated oven for 20-25 minutes, or until the cheese is melted and bubbly.
7. Serve the veggie enchiladas warm, with any desired toppings like diced avocado, sour cream, or chopped cilantro.

Storage Instructions:
Leftover veggie enchiladas can be stored in an airtight container in the refrigerator for up to 3 days. Reheat in the oven or microwave before serving.

Nutrition Information:
Calories: 400 | Protein: 18g | Carbohydrates: 52g | Fat: 15g | Saturated Fat: 6g | Cholesterol: 30mg | Sodium: 800mg | Fiber: 9g | Sugar: 6g

Dinner (23 Recipes)

92. Meatloaf with Mixed Veggies

Ingredients:
Meatloaf:
- 1 lb ground beef
- 1 cup breadcrumbs
- 1 egg
- 1/2 cup milk
- 1 onion, diced
- 2 cloves garlic, minced
- 1 teaspoon dried oregano
- 1/2 teaspoon salt
- 1/4 teaspoon black pepper

Veggie Medley:
- 2 carrots, peeled and diced
- 1 cup broccoli florets
- 1 cup cauliflower florets
- 1 cup green beans, trimmed and cut into 1-inch pieces
- 2 tablespoons olive oil
- 1/4 teaspoon salt
- 1/8 teaspoon black pepper

Equipment:
- Loaf pan
- Baking sheet
- Mixing bowl
- Knife and cutting board

Directions:
Meatloaf:
1. Preheat your oven to 375°F.
2. In a large mixing bowl, combine the ground beef, breadcrumbs, egg, milk, diced onion, minced garlic, dried oregano, salt, and black pepper. Mix until well incorporated.
3. Transfer the meatloaf mixture to a loaf pan and shape it into a loaf.
4. Bake the meatloaf in the preheated oven for 50-60 minutes, or until it reaches an internal temperature of 165°F.
5. Let the meatloaf rest for 5-10 minutes before slicing and serving.

Veggie Medley:
1. While the meatloaf is baking, toss the diced carrots, broccoli florets, cauliflower florets, and green bean pieces with the olive oil, salt, and black pepper on a baking sheet.
2. Roast the vegetables in the oven for 20-25 minutes, or until they are tender and lightly browned.

PreparationTime: 20 minutes
Cook Time: 1 hour
Total Time: 1 hour 20 minutes
Serves: 4

Nutrition Information:
Meatloaf:
Calories: 320 | Protein: 25g | Carbohydrates: 15g | Fat: 17g | Saturated Fat: 6g | Cholesterol: 120mg | Sodium: 550mg | Fiber: 1g | Sugar: 3g

Veggie Medley:
Calories: 120 | Protein: 4g | Carbohydrates: 12g | Fat: 7g | Saturated Fat: 1g | Cholesterol: 0mg | Sodium: 250mg | Fiber: 4g | Sugar: 4g

Dinner (23 Recipes)

93. Teriyaki Chicken with Rice

Ingredients:
Teriyaki Chicken:
- 1 lb boneless, skinless chicken breasts, cut into 1-inch cubes
- 1/2 cup teriyaki sauce
- 1 tablespoon honey
- 1 teaspoon sesame oil
- 1 clove garlic, minced
- 1/4 teaspoon ground ginger

Rice:
- 1 cup uncooked white rice
- 2 cups chicken broth or water

Equipment:
- Large skillet or wok
- Saucepan
- Cutting board and knife

PreparationTime: 15 minutes
Cook Time: 25 minutes
Total Time: 40 minutes
Serves: 4

Nutrition Information:

Teriyaki Chicken:
Calories: 220 | Protein: 27g | Carbohydrates: 10g | Fat: 7g | Saturated Fat: 1g | Cholesterol: 70mg | Sodium: 650mg | Fiber: 0g | Sugar: 8g

Directions:
Teriyaki Chicken:
1. In a large skillet or wok, combine the cubed chicken, teriyaki sauce, honey, sesame oil, minced garlic, and ground ginger.
2. Cook the chicken over medium-high heat, stirring occasionally, for 15-20 minutes, or until the chicken is cooked through and the sauce has thickened.

Rice:
1. In a saucepan, combine the uncooked white rice and chicken broth (or water).
2. Bring the mixture to a boil, then reduce the heat to low, cover, and simmer for 15-20 minutes, or until the rice is tender and the liquid is absorbed.

Serving: Serve the teriyaki chicken over the cooked rice.

Storage Instructions:
Leftover teriyaki chicken and rice can be stored separately in airtight containers in the refrigerator for up to 3 days. Reheat the chicken and rice before serving.

Tips:
- Encourage your 9-year-old to help with the preparation, such as measuring the ingredients or stirring the chicken in the skillet.
- Serve the teriyaki chicken and rice with a side of steamed broccoli or a fresh salad for a balanced meal.
- For a fun presentation, you can serve the teriyaki chicken and rice in a pineapple half or a hollowed-out bell pepper. - Adjust the amount of teriyaki sauce or honey to suit your child's taste preferences.

Dinner (23 Recipes)

94. Chocolate Chip Cookies

Ingredients:
- 2 1/4 cups all-purpose flour
- 1 teaspoon baking soda
- 1 teaspoon salt
- 1 cup unsalted butter, softened
- 3/4 cup granulated sugar
- 3/4 cup packed brown sugar
- 1 teaspoon vanilla extract
- 2 large eggs
- 2 cups semi-sweet chocolate chips

Equipment:
- Mixing bowls
- Hand mixer or stand mixer
- Baking sheets
- Parchment paper
- Cooling rack

PreparationTime: 15 minutes
Chill Time: 30 minutes
Bake Time: 10-12 minutes
Total Time: 55 minutes
Yields: 24 cookies

Nutrition Information:
Calories: 170 | Protein: 2g | Carbohydrates: 22g | Fat: 9g | Saturated Fat: 5g | Cholesterol: 25mg | Sodium: 125mg | Fiber: 1g | Sugar: 13g

Directions:
1. In a medium bowl, whisk together the flour, baking soda, and salt. Set aside.
2. In a large bowl, beat the softened butter, granulated sugar, and brown sugar with a hand mixer or stand mixer until light and fluffy, about 2-3 minutes.
3. Beat in the vanilla extract and then the eggs one at a time, mixing well after each addition.
4. Gradually add the dry ingredients to the wet ingredients, mixing just until combined. Fold in the chocolate chips.
5. Cover the dough and chill in the refrigerator for at least 30 minutes (or up to 3 days).
6. Preheat your oven to 375°F. Line baking sheets with parchment paper.
7. Scoop the chilled dough by the tablespoonful and place them about 2 inches apart on the prepared baking sheets.
8. Bake for 10-12 minutes, or until the edges are lightly golden brown.
9. Allow the cookies to cool on the baking sheets for 5 minutes before transferring them to a cooling rack.

Storage Instructions: Store the cooled cookies in an airtight container at room temperature for up to 1 week.

Tips:
- Encourage your 9-year-old to help with the preparation, such as measuring the ingredients, mixing the dough, or scooping the cookies onto the baking sheets.
- For a fun twist, let your child add their favorite mix-ins, like chopped nuts, M&Ms, or sprinkles.
- Serve the cookies with a cold glass of milk or a scoop of vanilla ice cream for a special treat.
- Adjust the baking time as needed, depending on the size of your cookies and your oven.

Baking (23 Recipes)

95. Vanilla Cupcakes with Sprinkles

Ingredients:
Cupcakes:
- 1 3/4 cups all-purpose flour
- 1 teaspoon baking powder
- 1/4 teaspoon salt
- 1/2 cup unsalted butter, softened
- 1 cup granulated sugar
- 2 large eggs
- 1 teaspoon vanilla extract
- 1/2 cup milk

Frosting:
- 1/2 cup unsalted butter, softened
- 3 cups confectioners' sugar
- 2-3 tablespoons heavy cream or milk
- 1 teaspoon vanilla extract
- Assorted sprinkles

Equipment:
- Cupcake tin with liners
- Mixing bowls
- Hand mixer or stand mixer
- Piping bag (optional)
- Offset spatula or butter knife

PreparationTime: 20 minutes
Bake Time: 18-20 minutes
Total Time: 40 minutes
Yields: 12 cupcakes

Frosting:
1. In a large bowl, beat the softened butter with a hand mixer or stand mixer until smooth and creamy.
2. Gradually add the confectioners' sugar, 1 cup at a time, beating well after each addition.
3. Add the heavy cream (or milk) and vanilla extract, and beat until the frosting is light and fluffy.

Assembly:
1. Once the cupcakes are completely cooled, use a piping bag or an offset spatula to frost the tops of the cupcakes.
2. Generously sprinkle the frosted cupcakes with assorted sprinkles.

Directions:
Cupcakes:

1. Preheat your oven to 350°F. Line a 12-cup cupcake tin with paper liners.

2. In a medium bowl, whisk together the flour, baking powder, and salt. Set aside.

3. In a large bowl, beat the softened butter and granulated sugar with a hand mixer or stand mixer until light and fluffy, about 2-3 minutes.

4. Beat in the eggs one at a time, then stir in the vanilla extract.

5. Alternate adding the dry ingredients and milk to the butter mixture, mixing just until combined after each addition.

6. Divide the batter evenly among the prepared cupcake liners, filling them about 3/4 full.

7. Bake for 18-20 minutes, or until a toothpick inserted into the center comes out clean.

8. Allow the cupcakes to cool in the tin for 5 minutes, then transfer them to a wire rack to cool completely.

Baking (23 Recipes)

96. Brownies

Ingredients:
- 1/2 cup (1 stick) unsalted butter, melted
- 1 cup granulated sugar
- 2 large eggs
- 1 teaspoon vanilla extract
- 1/3 cup all-purpose flour
- 1/4 cup unsweetened cocoa powder
- 1/4 teaspoon salt
- 1 cup semi-sweet chocolate chips

PreparationTime: 15 minutes
Bake Time: 25-30 minutes
Total Time: 40-45 minutes
Yields: 16 brownies

Equipment:
- 8x8 inch baking pan
- Mixing bowls
- Whisk or hand mixer
- Parchment paper (optional)

Directions:
1. Preheat your oven to 350°F. Grease an 8x8 inch baking pan or line it with parchment paper.
2. In a medium bowl, whisk together the melted butter and granulated sugar until combined.
3. Beat in the eggs one at a time, then stir in the vanilla extract.
4. In a separate bowl, whisk together the flour, cocoa powder, and salt.
5. Gradually add the dry ingredients to the wet ingredients, mixing just until combined. Fold in the chocolate chips.
6. Spread the brownie batter evenly into the prepared baking pan.
7. Bake for 25-30 minutes, or until a toothpick inserted into the center comes out with a few moist crumbs.
8. Allow the brownies to cool completely in the pan before cutting into squares.

Storage Instructions:
Store the cooled brownies in an airtight container at room temperature for up to 4 days.

Tips:
- Encourage your 9-year-old to help with the preparation, such as measuring the ingredients, mixing the batter, or sprinkling the chocolate chips.
- For a fun twist, let your child add their favorite mix-ins, like chopped nuts, peanut butter chips, or crushed candy.
- Serve the brownies with a scoop of vanilla ice cream or a drizzle of chocolate sauce for a special treat.
- Adjust the baking time as needed, depending on the size of your baking pan and your oven.

Nutrition Information:
Calories: 180 | Protein: 2g | Carbohydrates: 23g | Fat: 10g | Saturated Fat: 6g | Cholesterol: 35mg | Sodium: 55mg | Fiber: 1g | Sugar: 16g

Baking (23 Recipes)

97. Lemon Bars

Ingredients:
Crust:
- 1 cup (2 sticks) unsalted butter, softened
- 1/2 cup granulated sugar
- 2 cups all-purpose flour
- 1/4 teaspoon salt

Lemon Filling:
- 4 large eggs
- 1 1/2 cups granulated sugar
- 1/3 cup all-purpose flour
- 1/4 cup fresh lemon juice (about 2-3 lemons)
- 1 tablespoon grated lemon zest

Equipment:
- 9x13 inch baking pan
- Mixing bowls
- Hand mixer or stand mixer
- Parchment paper (optional)
- Sifter or fine-mesh strainer

Directions:
Crust:
1. Preheat your oven to 350°F. Grease a 9x13 inch baking pan or line it with parchment paper.
2. In a large bowl, beat the softened butter and granulated sugar with a hand mixer or stand mixer until light and fluffy.
3. Gradually add the flour and salt, mixing just until the dough comes together.
4. Press the dough evenly into the prepared baking pan.
5. Bake for 20-25 minutes, or until the crust is lightly golden.

Lemon Filling:
1. In a medium bowl, whisk together the eggs, granulated sugar, and flour until smooth.
2. Stir in the fresh lemon juice and lemon zest.
3. Pour the lemon filling over the baked crust.
4. Bake for an additional 10-15 minutes, or until the filling is set.
5. Allow the lemon bars to cool completely in the pan.
6. Once cooled, use a sifter or fine-mesh strainer to dust the top of the bars with confectioners' sugar.
7. Cut the lemon bars into squares and serve.

Storage Instructions:
Store the cooled lemon bars in an airtight container in the refrigerator for up to 5 days.

PreparationTime: 20 minutes
Bake Time: 30-35 minutes
Total Time: 55-60 minutes
Yields: 16 bars

Baking (23 Recipes)

98. Oatmeal Raisin Cookies

Ingredients:
- 1 cup (2 sticks) unsalted butter, softened
- 1 cup packed brown sugar
- 1 egg
- 1 teaspoon vanilla extract
- 1 1/2 cups all-purpose flour
- 1 teaspoon baking soda
- 1/2 teaspoon ground cinnamon
- 1/4 teaspoon salt
- 3 cups old-fashioned oats
- 1 cup raisins

PreparationTime: 15 minutes
Chill Time: 30 minutes
Bake Time: 10-12 minutes
Total Time: 55 minutes
Yields: 24 cookies

Equipment:
- Mixing bowls
- Hand mixer or stand mixer- Baking sheets
- Parchment paper- Cooling rack

Directions:
1. In a large bowl, beat the softened butter and brown sugar with a hand mixer or stand mixer until light and fluffy, about 2-3 minutes.
2. Beat in the egg and vanilla extract until combined.
3. In a separate bowl, whisk together the flour, baking soda, cinnamon, and salt.
4. Gradually add the dry ingredients to the wet ingredients, mixing just until combined. Fold in the old-fashioned oats and raisins.
5. Cover the dough and chill in the refrigerator for at least 30 minutes (or up to 3 days).
6. Preheat your oven to 350°F. Line baking sheets with parchment paper.
7. Scoop the chilled dough by the tablespoonful and place them about 2 inches apart on the prepared baking sheets.
8. Bake for 10-12 minutes, or until the edges are lightly golden brown.
9. Allow the cookies to cool on the baking sheets for 5 minutes before transferring them to a cooling rack.

Storage Instructions: Store the cooled cookies in an airtight container at room temperature for up to 1 week.

Tips:
- Encourage your 9-year-old to help with the preparation, such as measuring the ingredients, mixing the dough, or scooping the cookies onto the baking sheets.
- For a fun twist, let your child add their favorite mix-ins, like chopped nuts, chocolate chips, or dried cranberries.
- Serve the cookies with a glass of milk or a scoop of vanilla ice cream for a special treat.
- Adjust the baking time as needed, depending on the size of your cookies and your oven.

Baking (23 Recipes)

99. Chocolate Cake

Ingredients:
- 2 cups (250g) all-purpose flour
- 2 cups (400g) granulated sugar
- 3/4 cup (90g) unsweetened cocoa powder
- 1 1/2 teaspoons baking soda
- 1/2 teaspoon baking powder
- 1/2 teaspoon salt
- 2 large eggs
- 1 cup (240ml) milk
- 1/2 cup (120ml) vegetable oil
- 1 teaspoon vanilla extract
- 1 cup (240ml) boiling water

PreparationTime: 20 minutes
Cook Time: 30-35 minutes
Total Time: 50-55 minutes
Serves: 8-10

Equipment:
- 9-inch round baking pans (2)
- Mixing bowls
- Electric mixer
- Spatula
- Whisk

Directions:
1. Preheat the oven to 350°F (177°C). Grease and flour two 9-inch round baking pans.
2. In a large bowl, whisk together the flour, sugar, cocoa powder, baking soda, baking powder, and salt.
3. In a separate bowl, beat the eggs. Then add the milk, oil, and vanilla extract, and mix until well combined.
4. Slowly add the wet ingredients to the dry ingredients and mix on medium speed until just combined. Carefully stir in the boiling water. The batter will be thin.
5. Divide the batter evenly between the prepared baking pans.
6. Bake for 30-35 minutes, or until a toothpick inserted into the center comes out clean.
7. Allow the cakes to cool in the pans for 10 minutes, then remove them from the pans and let them cool completely on a wire rack.

Storage Instructions:
- Store the cooled cake layers in an airtight container at room temperature for up to 5 days.
- The cake can also be frozen for up to 3 months. Thaw at room temperature before serving.

Tips:
- For a richer chocolate flavor, use dark cocoa powder instead of unsweetened.
- To make a layered cake, spread frosting between the two cake layers and on the top and sides.
- Serve the cake with a scoop of vanilla ice cream or a dollop of whipped cream for an extra special treat.

Baking (23 Recipes)

100. Blueberry Scones

Ingredients:
- 2 cups (250g) all-purpose flour
- 1/4 cup (50g) granulated sugar
- 2 teaspoons baking powder
- 1/4 teaspoon salt
- 6 tablespoons (85g) unsalted butter, cold and cubed
- 3/4 cup (180ml) cold milk
- 1 cup (150g) fresh or frozen blueberries

PreparationTime: 15 minutes
Cook Time: 15-18 minutes
Total Time: 30-33 minutes
Serves: 8 scones

Equipment:
- Large mixing bowl
- Pastry cutter or two forks
- Baking sheet
- Parchment paper
- Knife or pizza cutter

Directions:
1. Preheat the oven to 400°F (204°C). Line a baking sheet with parchment paper.
2. In a large bowl, whisk together the flour, sugar, baking powder, and salt.
3. Cut in the cold butter using a pastry cutter or two forks until the mixture resembles coarse crumbs.
4. Gently fold in the blueberries.
5. Pour in the cold milk and stir just until a shaggy dough forms. Do not overmix.
6. Turn the dough out onto a lightly floured surface and gently knead it a few times.
7. Pat the dough into a 1-inch thick round. Cut into 8 wedges and place them on the prepared baking sheet.
8. Bake for 15-18 minutes, or until the tops are lightly golden brown.
9. Allow the scones to cool on the baking sheet for 5 minutes before serving.

Storage Instructions:
- Store the cooled scones in an airtight container at room temperature for up to 3 days.
- You can also freeze the baked scones for up to 3 months. Thaw at room temperature before serving.

Tips:
- For extra tender scones, use cold butter and cold milk.
- Avoid overmixing the dough, as this can make the scones tough.
- Serve the scones warm, with a pat of butter or a drizzle of honey.
- Let the 9-year-old girl help with mixing the dough and cutting the scones for a fun baking activity.

Nutrition Information: Calories | Carbohydrates | Protein | Fat | Saturated Fat | Cholesterol | Sodium | Fiber

Baking (23 Recipes)

101. Banana Bread

Ingredients:
- 1 3/4 cups (220g) all-purpose flour
- 1 teaspoon baking soda
- 1/4 teaspoon salt
- 1/2 cup (115g) unsalted butter, softened
- 3/4 cup (150g) granulated sugar
- 2 large eggs
- 1 teaspoon vanilla extract
- 1 1/4 cups (300g) mashed ripe bananas (about 3 medium bananas)

PreparationTime: 15 minutes
Cook Time: 55-60 minutes
Total Time: 1 hour 10 minutes - 1 hour 15 minutes
Serves: 8-10 slices

Equipment:
- Loaf pan (9x5 inches)
- Mixing bowls
- Electric mixer or hand mixer
- Spatula
- Toothpick or skewer

Directions:
1. Preheat the oven to 350°F (177°C). Grease and flour a 9x5 inch loaf pan.
2. In a medium bowl, whisk together the flour, baking soda, and salt.
3. In a large bowl, beat the butter and sugar together until light and fluffy, about 2-3 minutes.
4. Beat in the eggs one at a time, then stir in the vanilla and mashed bananas until well combined.
5. Gradually add the dry ingredients to the wet ingredients, mixing just until incorporated. Do not overmix.
6. Pour the batter into the prepared loaf pan and smooth the top.
7. Bake for 55-60 minutes, or until a toothpick inserted in the center comes out clean.
8. Allow the banana bread to cool in the pan for 10 minutes, then transfer to a wire rack to cool completely.

Storage Instructions:
- Store the cooled banana bread in an airtight container at room temperature for up to 4 days.
- You can also freeze the bread for up to 3 months. Thaw at room temperature before serving.

Tips:
- Use very ripe, spotty bananas for the best flavor.
- Let the 9-year-old girl help mash the bananas and mix the batter.
- Serve the banana bread with a smear of butter or a drizzle of honey for a tasty treat.
- For a fun twist, add chocolate chips, chopped nuts, or a streusel topping.

Baking (23 Recipes)

102. Peanut Butter Cookies

Ingredients:
- 1 cup (250g) creamy peanut butter
- 1 cup (200g) granulated sugar
- 1 large egg
- 1 teaspoon vanilla extract
- 1/4 teaspoon salt

PreparationTime: 10 minutes
Cook Time: 10-12 minutes
Total Time: 20-22 minutes
Serves: 18 cookies

Equipment:
- Mixing bowl
- Spoon or electric mixer
- Baking sheet
- Parchment paper
- Fork

Directions:

1. Preheat the oven to 350°F (177°C). Line a baking sheet with parchment paper.

2. In a medium bowl, combine the peanut butter, sugar, egg, vanilla, and salt. Mix until well blended.

3. Scoop the dough by the tablespoonful and place them about 2 inches apart on the prepared baking sheet.

4. Use a fork to gently press down on each cookie, creating a criss-cross pattern on the top.

5. Bake for 10-12 minutes, or until the cookies are lightly golden around the edges.

6. Allow the cookies to cool on the baking sheet for 5 minutes before transferring them to a wire rack to cool completely.

Storage Instructions:
- Store the cooled cookies in an airtight container at room temperature for up to 1 week.

- You can also freeze the cookies for up to 3 months. Thaw at room temperature before serving.

Tips:
- Let the 9-year-old girl help scoop the dough and press the fork pattern on the cookies.

- For extra peanut butter flavor, use crunchy peanut butter instead of creamy.

- Add a few chocolate chips or chopped peanuts to the dough for a fun twist.

- Serve the cookies with a cold glass of milk for a classic pairing.

Baking (23 Recipes)

103. Carrot Cake Muffins

Ingredients:
- 1 1/2 cups (190g) all-purpose flour
- 1 teaspoon baking powder
- 1/2 teaspoon baking soda
- 1/4 teaspoon salt
- 1 teaspoon ground cinnamon
- 1/2 cup (115g) unsalted butter, melted and slightly cooled
- 3/4 cup (150g) granulated sugar
- 2 large eggs
- 1 teaspoon vanilla extract
- 1 1/2 cups (150g) grated carrots (about 3 medium carrots)

Equipment:
- Muffin tin
- Cupcake liners
- Mixing bowls
- Whisk
- Grater
- Spoon or ice cream scoop

Directions:
1. Preheat the oven to 375°F (190°C). Line a 12-cup muffin tin with cupcake liners.
2. In a medium bowl, whisk together the flour, baking powder, baking soda, salt, and cinnamon.
3. In a separate large bowl, whisk together the melted butter, sugar, eggs, and vanilla until well combined.
4. Fold the dry ingredients into the wet ingredients until just combined. Gently fold in the grated carrots.
5. Scoop the batter into the prepared muffin cups, filling them about 3/4 full.
6. Bake for 18-20 minutes, or until a toothpick inserted into the center comes out clean.
7. Allow the muffins to cool in the tin for 5 minutes, then transfer them to a wire rack to cool completely.

Storage Instructions:
- Store the cooled muffins in an airtight container at room temperature for up to 4 days.
- You can also freeze the muffins for up to 3 months. Thaw at room temperature before serving.

Tips:
- Let the 9-year-old girl help grate the carrots and scoop the batter into the muffin cups.
- For a fun twist, add chopped walnuts or pecans to the batter.
- Serve the muffins with a dollop of cream cheese frosting or a sprinkle of powdered sugar.
- These muffins make a great snack or breakfast for the 9-year-old girl.

PreparationTime: 15 minutes
Cook Time: 18-20 minutes
Total Time: 33-35 minutes
Serves: 12 muffins

Baking (23 Recipes)

104. Raspberry Thumbprint Cookies

Ingredients:
- 1 cup (230g) unsalted butter, softened
- 3/4 cup (150g) granulated sugar
- 1 large egg
- 1 teaspoon vanilla extract
- 2 1/4 cups (280g) all-purpose flour
- 1/4 teaspoon salt
- 1/2 cup (120ml) raspberry jam

PreparationTime: 20 minutes
Cook Time: 12-14 minutes
Total Time: 32-34 minutes
Serves: 18 cookies

Equipment:
- Mixing bowls
- Electric mixer or hand mixer
- Baking sheet
- Parchment paper
- Spoon or small melon baller

Directions:
1. Preheat the oven to 350°F (177°C). Line a baking sheet with parchment paper.
2. In a large bowl, beat the butter and sugar together until light and fluffy, about 2-3 minutes.
3. Beat in the egg and vanilla until well combined.
4. In a separate bowl, whisk together the flour and salt.
5. Gradually add the dry ingredients to the wet ingredients, mixing just until a dough forms.
6. Scoop the dough by the tablespoonful and roll each into a smooth ball.
7. Place the dough balls about 2 inches apart on the prepared baking sheet.
8. Use your thumb or the back of a spoon to make a small indentation in the center of each cookie.
9. Fill each indentation with about 1 teaspoon of raspberry jam.
10. Bake for 12-14 minutes, or until the cookies are lightly golden around the edges.
11. Allow the cookies to cool on the baking sheet for 5 minutes before transferring them to a wire rack to cool completely.

Storage Instructions:
- Store the cooled cookies in an airtight container at room temperature for up to 1 week.
- You can also freeze the cookies for up to 3 months. Thaw at room temperature before serving.

Tips:
- Let the 9-year-old girl help roll the dough into balls and make the thumbprint indentations.
- For a fun twist, use different flavors of jam, such as strawberry or blackberry.
- Sprinkle the cookies with a light dusting of powdered sugar before serving.
- These cookies make a great snack or dessert for the 9-year-old girl

Baking (23 Recipes)

105. Sugar Cookies with Icing

Ingredients:
Cookies:
- 2 3/4 cups (345g) all-purpose flour
- 1 teaspoon baking powder
- 1/2 teaspoon salt
- 1 cup (230g) unsalted butter, softened
- 1 1/2 cups (300g) granulated sugar
- 1 large egg
- 2 teaspoons vanilla extract

Icing:
- 2 cups (240g) powdered sugar
- 3-4 tablespoons milk
- Food coloring (optional)
- Sprinkles (optional)

Equipment:
- Mixing bowls
- Electric mixer or hand mixer
- Rolling pin
- Cookie cutters
- Baking sheets
- Parchment paper
- Piping bag or zip-top bag (for icing)

PreparationTime: 20 minutes
Chilling Time: 1 hour
Cook Time: 8-10 minutes
Total Time: 1 hour 28 minutes - 1 hour 30 minutes
Serves: 24 cookies

Directions:
1. In a medium bowl, whisk together the flour, baking powder, and salt. Set aside.
2. In a large bowl, beat the butter and sugar together until light and fluffy, about 2-3 minutes.
3. Beat in the egg and vanilla until well combined.
4. Gradually add the dry ingredients to the wet ingredients, mixing just until a dough forms.
5. Divide the dough in half, shape each half into a disk, wrap in plastic wrap, and refrigerate for at least 1 hour.
6. Preheat the oven to 350°F (177°C). Line baking sheets with parchment paper.
7. On a lightly floured surface, roll out the dough to 1/4-inch thickness. Use cookie cutters to cut out shapes.
8. Transfer the cookies to the prepared baking sheets, spacing them about 2 inches apart.
9. Bake for 8-10 minutes, or until the edges are lightly golden.
10. Allow the cookies to cool on the baking sheets for 5 minutes before transferring them to a wire rack to cool completely.
11. Make the icing: In a medium bowl, whisk together the powdered sugar and 3 tablespoons of milk until smooth. Add more milk as needed to reach the desired consistency.
12. Transfer the icing to a piping bag or zip-top bag and pipe or spread the icing onto the cooled cookies. Decorate with sprinkles, if desired.

Baking (23 Recipes)

Creating a cookbook specifically for a 9-year-old girl is not just about providing delicious recipes; it's about fostering a love for cooking, encouraging healthy eating habits, and building confidence in the kitchen. The collection of 115 dishes in this book is carefully curated to be fun, nutritious, and easy to prepare, catering to the tastes and interests of young girls.

From the wholesome breakfast recipes that kickstart the day with energy and joy, to the delightful snacks that provide quick and healthy bites, every recipe is designed to be approachable and enjoyable. The lunch and dinner sections offer a variety of balanced meals that introduce young cooks to diverse flavors and ingredients, making mealtime both exciting and educational. And let's not forget the baking section, where creativity meets deliciousness, allowing young bakers to experiment with sweet treats and develop their baking skills.

This cookbook is more than a collection of recipes; it's an invitation to explore the culinary world, discover new favorites, and create lasting memories in the kitchen. Cooking can be a wonderful bonding activity, and through these recipes, parents and children can share moments of joy and accomplishment.

As this young girl embarks on her culinary adventures, may this book inspire her to continue exploring, learning, and enjoying the art of cooking. Happy cooking!

www.ingramcontent.com/pod-product-compliance
Lightning Source LLC
Chambersburg PA
CBHW081552250726
48653CB00009B/3390